Recent Results in Cancer Research

Fortschritte der Krebsforschung

Progrès dans les recherches sur le cancer

45

Edited by

*V. G. Allfrey, New York · M. Allgöwer, Basel · K. H. Bauer, Heidelberg
I. Berenblum, Rehovoth · F. Bergel, Jersey · J. Bernard, Paris
W. Bernhard, Villejuif · N. N. Blokhin, Moskva · H. E. Bock, Tübingen
P. Bucalossi, Milano · A. V. Chaklin, Moskva
M. Chorazy, Gliwice · G. J. Cunningham, Richmond · M. Dargent, Lyon
G. Della Porta, Milano · P. Denoix, Villejuif · R. Dulbecco, La Jolla
H. Eagle, New York · E. Eker, Oslo · R. A. Good, New York
P. Grabar, Paris · H. Hamperl, Bonn · R. J. C. Harris, Salisbury
E. Hecker, Heidelberg · R. Herbeuval, Nancy · J. Higginson, Lyon
W. C. Hueper, Fort Myers · H. Isliker, Lausanne
J. Kieler, København · G. Klein, Stockholm · H. Koprowski, Philadelphia
L. G. Koss, New York · G. Martz, Zürich · G. Mathé, Villejuif
O. Mühlbock, Amsterdam · W. Nakahara, Tokyo · L. J. Old, New York
V. R. Potter, Madison · A. B. Sabin, Washington · S. Sachs, Rehovoth
E. A. Saxén, Helsinki · C. G. Schmidt, Essen · S. Spiegelman, New York
W. Szybalski, Madison · H. Tagnon, Bruxelles · R. M. Taylor, Toronto
A. Tissières, Genève · E. Uehlinger, Zürich · R. W. Wissler, Chicago
T. Yoshida, Tokyo*

Editor in chief
P. Rentchnick, Genève

P. Koldovsky

Carcinoembryonic Antigens

With 4 Figures

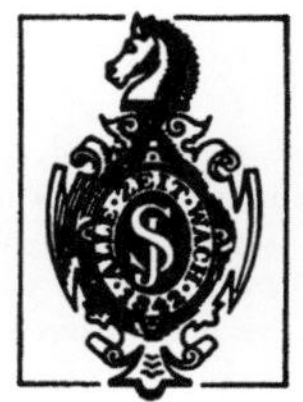

Springer-Verlag Berlin · Heidelberg · New York 1974

Pavel Koldovsky, M. D.
Research Department, The Children's Hospital of Philadelphia
1740 Bainbridge Street
Philadelphia

Sponsored by the Swiss League against Cancer

ISBN-13: 978-3-642-80812-8   e-ISBN-13: 978-3-642-80810-4
DOI: 10.1007/978-3-642-80810-4

Preface

Interest in the general field of tumor immunology has grown phenomenally in recent years. The number of publications continues to grow in seemingly exponential fashion and the end is not yet in sight. Under these conditions, it is very difficult for any individual investigator to perceive the whole, or even the small portion within which his own efforts must necessarily be confined. We are thus very fortunate when an investigator with long and wide experience in the field of tumor immunology takes the time to share his perspectives of a portion of that field. Dr. Koldovsky has been one of the pioneers in tumor immunology and he continues to contribute, especially in the area of CEA. In the present survey he has reviewed the status of CEA, setting forth not only the literature, but his own interpretation of that literature. For this endeavor, all workers in tumor immunology will be truely grateful.

November, 1973   R. T. Prehn

Contents

I. Introduction 1

II. Cell Membrane-Associated Antigens 2
   1. Immunity Against Cell Membrane-Associated Antigens 6

III. Antigenic Changes During Embryonic Development 11

IV. Tumor-Specific Antigens 19

V. Carcinoembryonic Antigens 24
   1. Cell-Surface CEA 24
   2. Alpha Fetoprotein 29
   3. Carcinoembryonic Antigens of the Digestive Tract 31
   4. As Yet Undefined Carcinoembryonic Antigens 34

VI. Properties of Carcinoembryonic Antigens 35
   1. Transplantation CEA 35
   2. Carcinoembryonic Antigens of the Liver Tumors — Alpha-Globulin . 36
   3. Carcinoembryonic Antigens of the Digestive Tract (GOLD) 38

VII. Clinical Significance of Carcinoembryonic Antigens 40
   1. Diagnostic and Prognostic Value 40
   2. Prospective Immunotherapeutic Uses of Carcinoembryonic Antigens . 49

VIII. Appendix: Methods of Detection, Separation and Purification of Carcinoembryonic Antigens 51
   1. Alpha Fetoprotein 51
   2. CEA of the Digestive Tract (GOLD) 53

IX. References 55

Subject Index 70

I. Introduction

The first attempts to cure cancer by immunologic means were made more than a century ago. Interest in tumor immunology has since increased, but there has been a certain degree of pessimism. TYZZER remarked in 1916 that reviewing the literature on tumor immunology was very difficult. In 1929 WOGLOM included almost 1000 references in his review and in 1942, SPENCER declared that the literature on tumor immunology was voluminous. However, positive results are reported much less frequently.

Tumors are an excellent tool for studying transplantation immunity and immuno-genetics. Using Japanese waltzing mice, LOEB (1901) discovered the strain specificity of tumor (tissue) transplantation. A few years later, FLEXNER and JOBLING (1907) described immunological enhancement of tumor transplants in rats preimmunized with heat-inactivated tumor tissue. Between 1916 and 1924, LITTLE and TYZZER (1924) found by means of tumor grafts that Mendelian inheritance applies to trans-plantation antigens. Tumors served as the tool of choise (BOLLAG, 1956) to detect immunological tolerance in heterologous relations. Tumor cells were also used to follow antigenic changes caused by mutation (BITTNER, 1935) or by growth in a histoincompatible but immunologically unreactive host (BARRETT, DERRINGER, 1959; MOLOMUT, 1960; MÖLLER, 1969; FELDMAN, 1963).

All of these studies are based on the assumption that the antigenic composition of normal and malignant tissues which originate from the same individual is identical. This assumption was proved to be valid by experiments in which successful immuni-zation against tumor grafts could be obtained with corresponding normal tissue (SCHONE, 1906). It was soon observed that immunization with embryonic tissue yielded better results than immunization with adult tissue. Since then, cross-reactivity between normal embryonic tissue and malignant tumors has been the subject in many experiments, and interest in the so-called carcinoembryonic (CEA) has increased in recent years. Studies of these antigens may be expected to lead to a better under-standing of the mechanism of malignant transformation and regulation of embryo-genesis. Practically speaking, they may prove to be valuable diagnostic, prognostic, and therapeutic aids.

That we all have been embryos and some of us will die of cancer is all that is certain about the relationship between cancer and embryonic antigens. What little is suspected above this level, I have presented in this book.

Questions concerning CEA are related to normal transplantation immunity, tolerance, enhancement, development of antigenicity and immunity during embryo-genesis, the mother fetus relationship and tumor-specific antigens. Therefore, the first three chapters are devoted to a brief summary of our knowledge in these areas.

II. Cell Membrane-Associated Antigens

Transplantation of tissues and organs is a widely used technique. It can be performed on the same organism (autotransplantation), between organisms of the same inbred strain (syngeneic graft), between members of a normal population (allogeneic graft) or between individuals of different species (hetero- or xenograft). In the beginning, all grafts look the same. Within a few days, however, a dramatic difference becomes apparent. Only the auto- and syngeneic grafts remain normal and of healthy appearance. The allo- and xenografts become inflamed: inflammation caused by the xenograft is usually more pronounced and appears sooner. Eventually both grafts form a hard crust and are rejected. The speed of the reaction is related to the relationship between the donor and the recipient. The farther the subjects are apart phylogenetically, the faster and stronger is the reaction.

Such reactions were observed at the end of the last century, not only with normal tissues but with malignant tumors as well. Eventually it was learned that this reaction is immunological in nature and that it is caused by differences in so-called transplantation antigens found in normal and malignant tissues.

Within a given population there are no two individuals so antigenically identical that they will retain skin grafts permanently. Monozygotic twins, however, are an exception to this rule. A second exception is inbred strains of animals, i.e., animals bred for many generations by brother-sister mating and selected for antigenic homogeneity. These syngeneic strains are primarily mice and rats, but guinea pigs, rabbits, hamsters, dogs, ducks and fish are also available. The uniqueness of a given individual in any randomly bred population, such as the human population is supposed to be, is guaranteed not by the existence of an unlimited number of individually specific transplantation antigens but rather by endless variation of a limited number of these antigens. This situation can be graphically illustrated by a simple schema (Fig. 1) of hypothetical population containing only five different antigens — A, B, C, D, E. In fact, each species must have more than a hundred such antigens. On this imaginary population individuum 1 will reject tissues from individuals 2 and 3 by reacting against antigen E. Individuum 3 will react against antigen A etc. In a situation with only five antigens and their possible combinations, individual specificity can be provided for 625 individuals; in the case of 100 such antigens, individual specificity can be provided for 100^{99} individuals, which is more than enough to assure individual specificity throughout the population, even for some generations at this rate of reproduction.

The transplantation antigens are expressed on the cell surface and in some form even on the endoplasmic reticulum (MANSON *et al.*, 1968). Only the antigens associated with the cell membrane, however, can be responsible for the transplantation reaction. Transplantation antigens are genetically controlled characteristics of the organism, and basically all cells of the same organism — both normal and malignant cells — contain the same set of such antigens. The inheritance of these antigens is controlled by Mendelian genetics (TYZZER and LITTLE, 1916, 1924). SNELL (1953) later formulated four main conditions which determine the fate of grafts:

1. Tumor isotransplants[1], i.e. tumors transplanted within the strain of origin grow progressively and kill all hosts.

2. Tumor homotransplants[2], i.e. tumor transplanted within the species but outside the strain of origin, fail to grow, or grow temporarily and then regress;

3. F_1 hybrids produced by crossing two inbred strain will grow tumor indigenous to either parent strain[3];

4. Only a fraction of mice of an F_2 generation, or of a backcross produced by mating to the resistant parent, will grow tumors from the inbred lines involved.

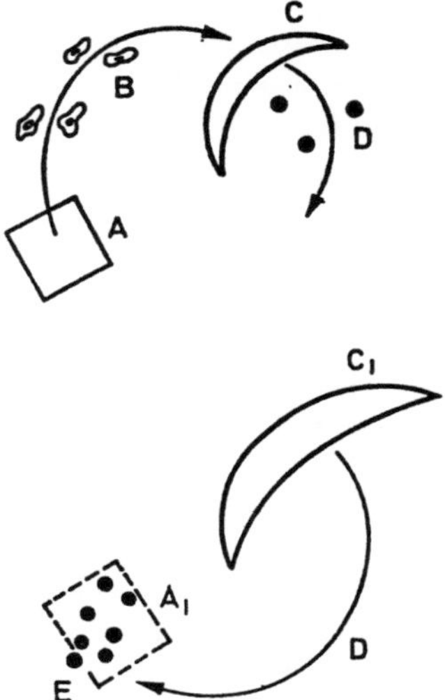

Fig. 1. Immunological reaction expressed in the form of a reflex arc. Initial the antigenic stimulus (A) (skin graft) is recognized as foreign and information about it is carried by afferent way (B) (macrophages?) to immunological centrum (C) (spleen, lymph nodes). Here are produced antibodies and immune cells and carried efferently (D) to the target (foreign skin graft). Finally, the graft destroyed by immune cells (E) (small lymphocytes)

The transplantation antigens can be divided according to their "strength", i.e. the speed and strength of the transplantation reaction they are able to elicit. This phenomenon has been studied most extensively in mice. The "strong" antigens elicit skin-graft rejection within 10—12 days and the "weak" antigens cause a reaction within 14 or more days. In some strain combinations, the reaction takes up to several months. In every species, several genetic loci occur on the chromosomes on which

---

1 Current terminology: syngeneic.
2 Current terminology: allogenic.
3 Animals of both parent strains will reject tumors derived from F_1 hybrids.

are located genes which control the expression of these antigens. IVANYI (1970) summarized knowledge about these loci. It is interesting to note that in every species, several loci (small loci) control the less important antigens and one major locus controls the most important antigens (e.g. H-2 locus in mice). This major locus, also known as the major histocompatibility locus, is linked to a chromosomal region which represents a major gene for reproductive performance. SNELL (1968) pointed out that both systems form a unit (super gene).

In addition to transplantation antigens, which are characteristic for a given species and individuum, (or whole population of an inbred strain) other antigens belonging to the different groups are found on the cell membrane. One group includes the organ (tissue-)specific antigens. Specific antigens have been detected in: brain, thyroid, testis, lens of the eye, kidney, liver, pancreas. Under pathological conditions these antigens can elicit an autoimmune reaction which leads to damage or even to destruction of a given organ. It is probable that almost every organ (tissue) has its own specific antigen. They have not yet been detected since no-one has really looked for them. In recent years, this point was nicely illustrated with cells belonging to the same tissue — peripheral white blood cells. RAFF (1970) showed that white blood cells can be divided according to their antigenic properties into T (thymus-dependent) and B (bone marrow-derived) cells. These cells also differ in their functional capacity: the T cells are responsible for cell-mediated immunity and the B cells, for antibody production.

The other antigens on the cell membrane are antigens specific for the male sex. They are controlled by the Y chromosome and are classified as "weak" antigens (like the previous ones). They cross-react within a given species, i.e., mice of different strain have the same Y-linked antigen.

Other antigens which should be discussed in connection with the antigenic composition of the cell membrane are antigens which, under normal conditions, are not present on (or in) the cell membrane of a healthy cell. These antigens can be either extracellular products (proteins) of the cell itself or pathologic organisms coming from the outside (bacteria, PPLO, viruses). The first group includes a large variety of cell products — enzymes, hormones, intermediate metabolic products. Our knowledge of their potential influence on the immunological properties of the cell and of the reaction of the organism against them is almost nil. Two such extracellular antigens — both CEA — will be discussed later (p. 24 and 27).

For many reasons, the members of the second group responsible for cell membrane-associated antigen changes, i.e. microorganisms, are also very important. Viruses which are released from the cell by budding through the cell membrane are, for a certain period of time, really a part of the cell membrane. It was demonstrated for certain budding viruses (e.g. rabies, SV_5; WIKTOR et al., 1968) that neutralizing antibodies can be cytotoxic for virus-infected and virus-producing cells. Mycoplasma are another example of organisms closely related to the cell membrane. A relatively high proportion of the human population has antibodies against mycoplasma. Such antibodies can damage mycoplasma-infected cells. Even infection with much larger organisms, e.g., bacteria, can cause changes in the antigenic composition of the cell membrane. Sympathetic ophthalmia is a textbook example of such a situation. The retina of one eye is infected by bacteria against which the organism begins to react immunologically. During this process the diseased organism begins to develop immunity against retina-specific antigens by first reacting against the cell membrane of the infected cells. In the last stage of the disease, the healthy (non-infected eye) is attacked by the autoimmune reaction. This development can be prevented by timely surgical removal of the infected eye.

The so-called tumor specific transplantation antigen (TSTA), which can be compared to the organ-tissue-specific antigen, has an interesting position among cell membrane-associated antigens. In tumors induced by oncogenic viruses, TSTA is common to any tumor induced by the same virus, regardless of the strain or species in which the tumor originated. In virus-induced, nonvirus-producing tumors, the TSTA is a true component of the cell membrane (a cell membrane antigenic change), and not directly part of the virus. In virus-induced tumors which produce virus, it is sometimes very difficult to distinguish between the antivirus and anti-TSTA reaction. This problem is encountered primarily in the virus-induced leukemias. In a situation in which nononcogenic viruses are suspected of inducing cell membrane-associated antigenic changes, the presence of virus makes definitive demonstration of such an antigen very difficult (ROIZMAN, 1965).

In addition to multiplying agents, e.g. viruses, bacteria and mycoplasma can be temporarily associated with the cell membrane and so simulate membrane antigens, proteins and carbohydrates, e.g. products of other cells or artificially added products, can also modify antigenic expression. Guinea-pig complement, which can be relatively firmly attached to the receptor on the cell membrane is an example of the latter; antibodies to guinea-pig complement will damage such cells.

This complement, which is passively transferred during cell multiplication and merely "diluted", remains attached to the cell for several generations. Thus anti-complement antibodies are still active in progeny of the complement-"infected" cells for several cell divisions (BORSOS *et al.*, 1970). Clinically important is a possible antigenic change of all surface by binding certain drugs (e.g. amidoyrin) to the surface of certain cells and many produce antigenic changes in the cell surface, a phenomenon which may be of clinical significance. In such cases, during prolonged administration, a patient can develop antibodies to these drugs, which can be cytotoxic for given cells. In addition, antibodies may utilize a certain drug to form an antigen-antibody complex which binds to the cell surface and renders the cell susceptible to complement-mediated lysis. Theoretically such induced antigenic changes could develop during anticancer treatment or, on the other hand, they could be used as an approach to anticancer immunity in man. In the latter situation, tumor cells obtained from the patient during an operation would first be antigenically modified by a particular drug. The patient would then be immunized against this drug and later injected with his own, nonrepopulating tumor cells which had also been antigenically modified with the same drug. The cells would then be destroyed by a secondary immunological reaction; in the meantime the organism would be immunized by TSTA released from the newly attacked cells. Finally, the malignant cells which were not removable by operation would be attacked immunologically. Unfortunately, such speculation, even though it is being considered by many people, is still far from practical realization.

Care should be taken in isolating antigenic preparations from cells. For example, if the antigen(s) of interest have protein components, use of proteolytic enzymes during processing may cause a change in the structure of the protein and hence a change in its antigenic properties. Similar problems arise with antigens such as neuraminidase if enzymes active against carbohydrate components are used. If the use of such enzymes cannot be avoided, appropriate controls should be done using mechanical disruption of the cells.

From the point of view of antitumor immunity, such as transplantation immunity, important changes can be caused by an intrinsic factor within a given cell population. Like all genetically controlled characteristics, antigens can be changed by mutation (BITTNER, 1935). The mutation rate of transplantation antigens in certain strains of mice is surprisingly high (Genetics Conference, The Hague, 1964). Another possible antigenic change is the so-called antigenic modification which can be caused by several mechanisms. It was observed that the antigenic expression of a tumor could be changed after growth in an antigenically incompatible (not identical) host, which for some reason did not react against the allograft (e.g., for tumors grafted in immunologically enhanced hosts, see MOLOMUT, 1958; in F_1 hybrids, BARRET and DERRINGER, 1950; in newborn or heavily irradiated animals, FELDMAN and SACHS, 1957). Some antigenic modifications can occur even within normal skin grafts allografted to allogeneic but tolerant recipients. In our laboratory, we have shown that the TSTA of methylcholanthrene-induced tumors persists after repeated passages of very large doses of cells in mice resistant to a normal dose of tumor cells (KOLDOVSKY and SVOBODA, 1962). SJOGREN, 1964, found that even after 42 passages of a polyoma-induced tumor in animals immunized against polyoma TSTA, the polyoma TSTA was still detectable. It was recently demonstrated with ferritin-labelled antibodies that TSTA induced Gross virus disappears when the tumor is grown in a host which has received specific immune pressure, but reappears after growth in a normal, non-preimmunized host (AOKI and JOHNSON, 1972).

1. Immunity Against Cell Membrane-Associated Antigens

All of the cell membrane-associated antigens can elicit an immunological response, which can lead to the damage or destruction of the target cells, to immunological enhancement or to tolerance (immunological paralysis). Such immunological reactions can be viewed in terms of the reaction shown in Fig. 2. First comes the antigenic stimulus — by a cell which is antigenically incompatible with the host. Such cells are found and recognized as foreign by cells within the host which are specifically designed for this function — the macrophages. The macrophages — receptor information cells — carry this information to the immunological response centers, i.e., to the lymph nodes and spleen. Here they stimulate production of specific immune cells (and/or antibodies) — effector cells — which, travelling in an efferent direction, reach the target cells and destroy them. The effector cells are very similar to small lymphocytes. When an organism encounters for a second time foreign cells antigenically identical to those previously encountered, it responds with a so-called secondary immunological reaction. This response is faster and more vigorous, for example, if a skin graft is rejected by the primary response within about 12 days, the graft will be destroyed by the secondary response within 6 days. The memory for such a response is long and for some antigens, can last almost the entire lifetime of the given individual. This secondary response is specific: the

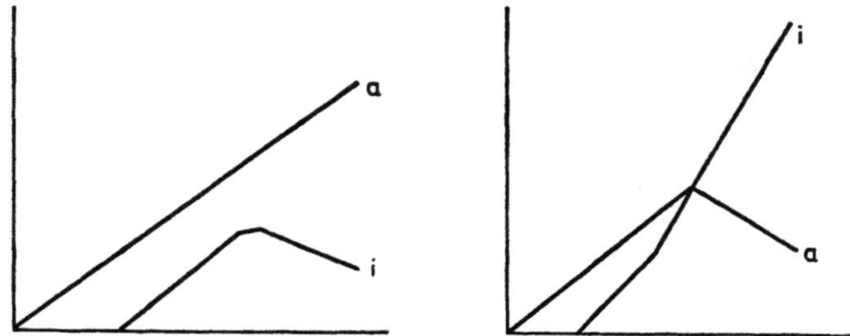

Fig. 2. Competition between tumor growth and development of immunity — in the first case the tumor growth is so fast that the immune apparatus of the host cannot destroy it. At the end of the tumor growth, the immune capacity of tumor-bearing organism can be exhausted (specifically or nonspecifically). In the second case, the organism is able to produce a sufficiently strong immunological reaction to destroy the tumor in time

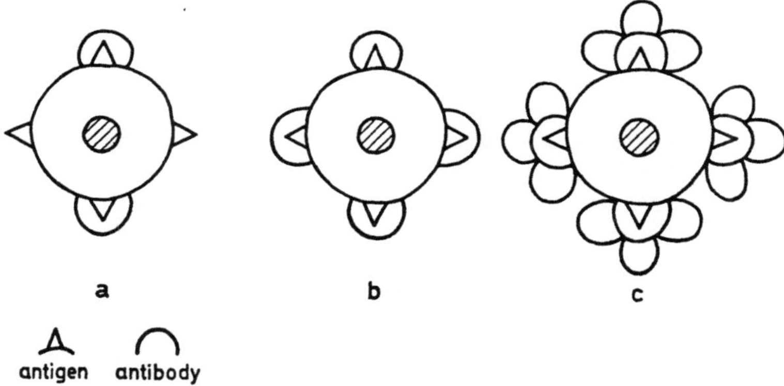

Fig. 3. Schematic expression of three quantitatively different ratios between antigen and antibodies and the consequent tumor growth. A: not all antigenic sites (determinant groups) are covered and the cell is still sensitive to action of immune cells. Such tumor can be finally rejected by immune cells. B: all antigens are coated and such a cell is protected against the action of immune cells. Such tumors can exhibit enhanced growth (immunological enhancement, blocking). C: excessive amount of antibodies are available; this can lead to direct destruction of tumor cells in the presence of complement

application of other foreign antigenically nonrelated cells elicits only a primary response. The immune reaction occurs under normal conditions when a certain amount of foreign tissue enters fully reactive host. It should also occur in response to normal cells which become transformed, develop TSTA and begin to exhibit the growth properties of a tumor. Such cells are eliminated to control such "spontaneous" malignancies. This hypothesis is supported both by experimental and by clinical observations. It was demonstrated that adult mice inoculated with doses of polyoma virus which do not cause a progressively growing tumor, were immune to subsequent grafts of polyoma tumors. The best explanation is that in the case of the virus-injected mice, a few cells were transformed by the virus but were recognized as foreign because of polyoma TSTA and were eliminated before they could start to form a malignant tumor. We can imagine such a situation as a race between the speed of tumor growth (cell division of the newly transformed cells) and the production of enough immune cells able to destroy the tumor cells. Several indirect clinical observations support the possibility that a similar situation exists in humans. For example, body fluids taken from wounds following an operation contain malignant cells more often than would be consistent with the percentage of patients with recurring tumors. These cells were somehow eliminated. In addition, microscopic carcinoma of the prostate without signs of progressive growth are found in biopsies of old men more often than would correspond with the incidence of this tumor (SOUTHAM, 1961).

Such reactions can unfortunately occur against one's own normal tissue and cause autoimmune disease. In the case of tumor growth, one would wish to encourage the immune reaction against the tumor, while in the case of autoimmune disease, the immune reaction should be suppressed, a goal which is shared by surgeons wishing to replace diseased or missing organs (tissues) by allografting.

Suppression (prevention) can be achieved nonspecifically — by drugs, irradiation, cortisone, antilymphocytic serum (HUMPHREY, 1971). We shall, however, discuss briefly the specific suppression of transplantation immunity: immunological tolerance and immunological enhancement.

Immunological enhancement has never been fully understood, though it has been known for more than half a century (FLEXNER and JOBLING, 1907). Animals specifically immunized with inactivated tumor cells (heat-inactivated, frozen, lyophilized) respond in a paradoxical way. When they are injected with transplanted living cells of the same tumor, growth of the tumor is accelerated or enhanced, rather than inhibited. This phenomenon is antigenically specific, and antigens associated with the cell membrane are responsible for it. Most likely, they are the same antigens as those which are responsible for the rejection reaction. The reaction is readily transferable by serum (cf. KALISS, 1956), though more easily by allogeneic serum than by heterologous serum. The phenomenon was demonstrated not only against normal transplantation antigens but also against tumor-specific transplantation antigens (BUBENIK and KOLDOVSKY, 1964; MÖLLER, 1964). Sometimes the enhancement can be transferred by immune cells still producing enhancing antibodies in the new host (KOLDOVSKY, 1969). Enhancement is not limited to tumors, but also occurs against transplants of normal tissue, where it is less easily detectable. When whole serum has the capacity to transfer enhancement, the 7 S fraction is several times more powerful than the 19 S fraction (KOLDOVSKY, 1969).

There are several theories concerning the mechanism of immunological enhancement. Part of the effect can be explained by "coating". The enhancing antibodies coat the antigenic determinant groups on the cell surface, against which they are directed. Such coating renders the cells nonrecognizable for the effector cells. The reaction seems to be dependent on the proportion of antigenic sites on the cell surface and on the number of available antibody molecules. For full effect all antigens should be coated (Fig. 4) (KOLDOVSKY, 1969).

The blocking phenomenon was also demonstrated *in vitro* (MÖLLER, 1964; HELLSTROM *et al.*, 1970). It was recently proposed that antigen antibody complexes are responsible for this blocking effect and that unblocking antibodies exist (SJOGREN *et al.*, 1971). These observations, however, do not exclude the possibility that some kind of central inhibition is also involved in immunological enhancement *in vivo*. Such a possibility provides a link between immunological enhancement and immunological tolerance, as originally proposed by VOISIN (1961) and discussed recently by the HELLSTRÖMS (1971).

The theory of immunological tolerance was proposed by BURNET and FENNER (1949). They speculated that new antigens which appear during embryogenesis are recognized by the developing immunological apparatus of the organism as "self" components. Against these antigens reactions should not take place later in life. If an antigen is artificially introduced in the organism during this developmental period and presented to the immunological apparatus as "own" material (BURNET's "self and nonself"), the immunological apparatus can be "fooled" so that subsequently it will not react to the same antigen. Thus, immunological tolerance is specific.

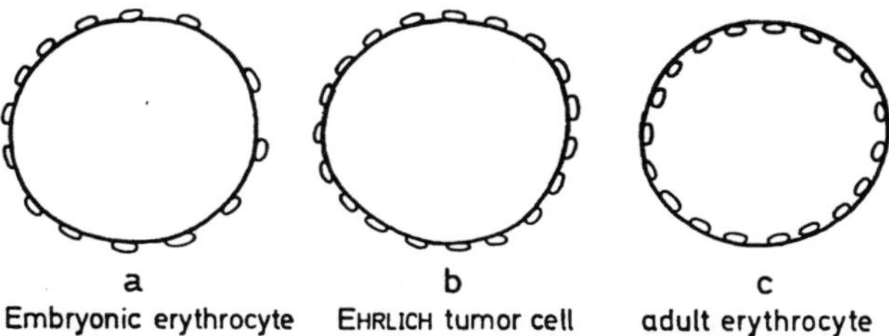

Fig. 4. Specific antigens (which crossreact) are expressed on the surface of the tumor cells and on embryonal erythrocytes, but on the inner side of the membrane of erythrocytes in the adult mouse

BILLINGHAM *et al.*, 1953, used two strains of mice to prove this theory for normal transplantation antigens. Near-term mouse embryos of one strain were injected *in utero* with spleen cells from another strain. When the embryos developed into immunologically mature animals, they tolerated skin grafts from the strain which donated the spleen cells but not from unrelated strains of mice.

At the same time HASEK (1953) was studying the speculation by Lysenko that inheritance is more dependent on external factors than on nuclear (chromosomal DNA) material. In experiments to produce genetic changes in birds after so-called vegetative hybridization, HASEK joined extraembryonal vessels of two developing chicken embryos (embryonic parabiosis). No genetic changes were observed, but the embryonic parabiotic partners did not react against each other immunologically. It was also observed that this induced nonreactivity was immunologically specific and, in the case of the same species (chicken), lasted the entire lifetime of the animals. Embryonic parabiosis later proved to be the most effective method for producing immunological tolerance; in fact, tolerance between individuals of two different species (chicken, turkey) can be obtained (HRABA, 1969). Natural parabiosis during embryonic life leading to immunological tolerance has also been described for cattle (OWEN, 1948), sheep (HRABA *et al.*, 1959), and marmosets.

It appears that the induction of specific immunological nonreactivity is not limited only to the period preceding birth, though the embryonic stage is the most suitable time to do so. When an excess amount of antigen is administered to an immunologically mature organism, immunological paralysis can result. For example, if a mouse which receives a dose of pneumococcal polysaccharide which is 1000 times higher than the optimal immunizing dose, the mouse is later unable to react against the bacteria (FELTON, 1954). It could also be shown for transplantation antigens (MARTINEZ *et al.*, 1962), and it is easier to induce paralysis with weak, i.e., phylogenetically closer, antigens. The paralyzing dose for some tumor-specific transplantation antigens is only 5—10 times higher than the optimal immunizing dose (KOLDOVSKY, 1969).

Immunological tolerance need not last the entire life of the organism. In newborn animals which receive injections of the antigen being studied, the experimentally induced tolerance often disappears within a few months. The tolerance can also be experimentally terminated by adoptive transfer of immunity or by immunization with cross-reactive antigens. This is important to keep in mind while discussing the possibility of an organism being tolerant to certain embryo-specific antigens and the question of permanence of tolerance. It is also important to know whether the organism is able to react later against these antigens when they appear as the result of malignant transformation.

Until now the discussion has been confined to antigens localized in or on the cell membrane. Intracellularly localized cell particles are also antigenic. These antigens can either be identical to some of the cell-membrane antigens (antigen of H-2 type on cell reticulum) or have their own specific antigenicity, nucleus, intracellularly localized virus and its subunits showing different antigenicity, enzymes, metabolic products, etc. From the point of view of tumors, the so-called complement-fixing antigens (T, GS antigens) which result from the interaction of an oncogenic virus with the cell are also of interest. They have been studied intensively and are the subject of several recent reviews. They will be discussed briefly later (p. 19).

Many extracellular products are also antigenic and have been studied from various points of views. They will be discussed later in connection with malignancy and its relation to the embryo. One extracellular product, antibodies themselves, is strongly antigenic and can have an important relationship to tumors and embryonic growth.

III. Antigenic Changes During Embryonic Development

The genetic material of an egg and a sperm contains the information for all of antigens which will appear under normal conditions during embryonic development and during the whole of the life of the organism. In the beginning, however, both cells seem to be very poor antigenically, the egg in particular. PALM *et al.* (1971) have shown that an unfertilized mouse egg and a very early mouse embryo — at the level of a few cells — show negative membrane-fluorescence staining with otherwise positive anti-H-2 serum. Antisera prepared against weak histocompatibility antigens (H-1, H-6) produced a positive membrane fluorescence reaction with the unfertilized egg, and the embryo at the level of a few cells. We recently reported (KOLDOVSKY *et al.*, 1972) that guinea-pig antiserum prepared against unfertilized mouse eggs is highly cytotoxic for these eggs, but such an antiserum has no detectable cytotoxic activity against normal mouse cells from an adult animal. Unfertilized mouse eggs are also insensitive to the cytotoxic action of guinea-pig antiserum to mouse spleen cells or to mouse anti-H-2 antigen antibodies. The effect of guinea-pig antisera against unfertilized mouse eggs seems to be species-specific (rat, hamster, rabbit). This property is different from that of organ-specific antigens, which usually cross the species barrier.

Sperms, although they are practically naked nuclei, have an antigenically richer surface. The presence of H-2 antigens on mouse spermatozoa can be demonstrated by several methods: by immunofluorescence (BARTH and RUSSEL, 1964; BECH *et al.*, 1962), by absorption of agglutinating antibodies (SNELL, 1944), and by induction of tolerance by sterile mating (PREHN, 1960). The presence of H-2, H-3, H-13, and Y-linked antigens can be shown by immunofluorescence, skingraft rejection, absorption of hemagglutinating antibodies (VOJTISKOVA *et al.*, 1969) and by cytotoxicity testing (GOLDBERG *et al.*, 1970). Transplantation antigens of the human system (HI-A) are expressed on human sperms (HAMERLYNCH and RUHMKE, 1968). The experiments of FELONS and DAUSSET (1970), indicate very strongly that sperms, as cells with a haploid number of chromosomes, have quantitatively a haploid expression of HL-A. The presence of the AB 0 blood-group antigen system, was demonstrated some time ago (LANDSTEINER and LEVINE, 1928). LEHRS (1930) and PUTHONEN (1930) found that people can be classified according to the presence of AB 0 antigens in the body fluids as secretors (body fluids are AB 0-antigen positive) and non-secretors (body fluids are negative). In recent work, FERNANDES *et al.* (1972) showed that human anti-A and anti-B sera do not agglutinate the corresponding human spermatozoa and have no cytotoxic or immobilizing activity for sperms. Sperms from a secretor absorb a higher proportion of anti-AB 0 antibodies than do red blood cells, even after being washed 10 times with saline. The expression of transplantation antigens on sperms, at least in chickens, is not so complete as on the surface of, say, spleen cells. HASEK (1959) could not induce tolerance against skin grafts in chickens using a pure suspension of sperms under conditions in which tolerance was inducible with spleen cells.

Besides the antigens common to most somatic cells, sperms contain organ- or tissue-specific antigens, as can be demonstrated by autoimmunization (LANDSTEINER, 1899; METCHNIKOFF, 1900; FREUND, 1953). The head contains antigens different from the rest of the spermatozoon (HENLE *et al.*, 1938). Relating to immune mechanisms involved in transplantation reactions and antitumor immunity is the interesting finding of CHUTNA and POKORNA (1967) and POKORNA (1970) that specific heterologous antisperm antibodies contain at least two fractions: IgM, which is cytotoxic for testicular cells and IgG, which exhibits protective activity. The immunological tolerance against sperm organ-specific antigen can prevent induction of auto-immune aspermatogenesis (VOJTISKOVA *et al.*, 1962).

When the sperm and ovum finally fuse, expression of normal transplantation antigens is still limited during the early stages of embryonic development. During the developmental period, however, the cell membrane-associated antigens undergo extensive quantitative and qualitative changes.

In the first hours and days, the developing embryo expresses almost as few transplantation antigens as the unfertilized egg itself. SIMMONS and RUSSEL (1962) transplanted fertilized mouse ova originating from the mating of two different strains beneath the renal capsule of mice of the maternal strain. The ova developed into agglomerates of trophoblastic cells which did not provoke a reaction against a subsequent skin graft derived from a paternal strain. Trophoblastic proliferation was not inhibited by previous immunization with paternal skin. In additional experiments, SIMMONS and RUSSEL (1965) transplanted ova of one strain (C 3 H mice), 1.5—2.5 days after coitus, to mice of another strain (C 5 7 Bl) hyperimmunized against the transplantation antigens of the strain of ova donors. Control, non-immunized allogeneic recipients supported the growth of such ova in the same way as syngeneic recipients (80% and 84%, respectively), but development was detectable in only 25% of the allogeneic recipients preimmunized with a single skin graft, and no growth was detectable in the hyperimmune recipients. Fertilized mouse ova can form trophoblast tumor-like masses even in a heterologous recipient (KIRBY, 1962; SIMMONS and RUSSEL, 1964). OLDS (1968) prepared eggs of the two-celled stage from Balb/c mice and removed the zona pellucida with pronase. Using the mixed agglutination reaction, she demonstrated the presence of H-2 antigens on the ova. EIDID (1964) demonstrated rejection of 9-day-old embryo tissue grafted onto a preimmunized adult host. ZEICH (1969) demonstrated that mice grafted with rat ova responded immunologically against them, but that the grafts still produced hormones which circulated in the heterologous host. CHUTNA and HASKOVA (1959) succeeded in inducing transplantation reaction against skin grafts by means of immunization with 8½-day mouse embryos. Detection of sensitivity against existing immunity or induction of resistance, however, indicates that some of the transplantation antigens are present, but is by no means a guarantee that all antigens are already fully expressed. The experiments mentioned above only show that mouse embryos in the very early stages of development already have some of the transplantation antigens which are expressed on the somatic cells of the adult organism; they do not indicate how complete this antigenic complement is. In this respect, experiments concerned with induced immunological tolerance should be more informative. For example, must a certain threshold amount of all of the major antigens be represented to induce tolerance to certain tissues? As far as I know, because of experimental difficulties, only one experiment has been done to study this. HASEK (1960) induced tolerance to allogeneic skin grafts in chickens by injecting newborn chicks with $4\frac{1}{2}$-day chicken embryos.

The surface antigens of developing embryos undergo dynamic changes. SCHLESINGER (1964) monitored the antigenicity of mouse embryonic and trophoblastic tissue by quantitative absorption of isohemagglutinins. The presence of H-2 isoantigen (alloantigen) was detected in the earliest embryos (C 3 H strain) studied ($10\frac{1}{2}$ day). The antigenicity of the liver increased rapidly between $13\frac{1}{2}$ and $15\frac{1}{2}$ days, after which the level remained constant. In preterm embryos, all of the antigens of the adult thymus are present: H-2 antigens were not detectable on trophoblasts of $2\frac{1}{2}$- and $3\frac{1}{2}$-day mouse ova. Similarly, DORIA (1963) demonstrated that liver from $13\frac{1}{2}$-day embryos did not induce immunity against corresponding skin grafts whereas liver from $15\frac{1}{2}$-day embryos did induce transplantation immunity.

That such results are not caused by the maturation of the transplantation antigens in embryonic tissue after grafting but by the presence of antigens already present at the time of grafting, was demonstrated by using heavily irradiated (nonrepopulating) embryonic tissue (TYAN and COLE, 1962; MÖLLER, 1963). However, the concentration of transplantation antigens gradually increases with the age of the embryo (BASH and STETSON, 1963; MÖLLER, 1963). MÖLLER (1960) studied the development of antigens of the H-2 system in newborn mice. Erythrocytes and spleen cells from C 3 H mice were not sensitive to anti-H-2 antibodies until 2—3 days after birth. Normal sensitivity was reached at the age of 6 days. Erythrocytes from C 3 H mice of less than $1\frac{1}{2}$ days old did not absorb anti-H-2 agglutinins *in vitro*, but spleen, liver and kidney cells already had this capacity.

The main purpose of the above-mentioned experiments was to demonstrate the presence of histocompatibility antigens in general, paying little attention to which locus controls these antigens. KLEIN showed that both the H-2 (1965a) and H-3 (1965b) antigens are already detectable in 12-day embryos.

Species other than mice are not as well defined antigenically, so less is known about antigenic changes during their embryonic development. Isoagglutinogens are present in 15-day rabbit embryos (MITCHISON, 1953). In rats, isoagglutinogens develop very rapidly during the first 14 days after birth and reach the level of an adult rat about two months after birth. In cattle, most red-cell isoantigens are probably present at birth. In humans, the HL-A or blood-group antigens are expressed long before birth; however, studies on very young embryos have not yet been done.

To understand the mother fetus relationship as an immunological problem and to consider the possibility of the reappearance of embryonic antigens during malignant transformation and of reactivity against them, it is important to know how the immunological apparatus develops during embryonic life, i.e., at what stage is the embryo able to recognize foreign antigens and to react against them, either by immunological tolerance or by immunity? Such questions are certainly more complicated than those about antigenic composition during various stages of embryonic development. The response to an antigen depends on two factors: 1) the phylogenetic "distance" between the host and the antigen, and 2) sometimes to a greater extent, the dose of the antigen. Extreme increase of the antigenic dose can induce immunological paralysis even in an adult, immunologically mature organism.

Theoretically one would assume that in the very early stages of development where no immune apparatus exists, introducing a new antigen would lead to no response neither to tolerance nor to immunity. Such experiments are difficult to perform in mammals. SIMMONSEN (1955) demonstrated in chickens that tolerance to human erythrocytes could be induced during the period between 14—19 days; earlier injection of human erythrocytes had no effect.

If the status of the immunological apparatus is considered in terms of the inducibility of tolerance, large differences can be seen among various species. The sheep fetus is probably the most immunologically mature, since it can reject a skin graft as early as one month before birth (SCHINKEL and FERGUSON, 1956). The donor of the rejected skin was the mother, indicating that the embryo is able to react against the mother's antigens. This fact represents an additional complication of the immunological relationship between the mother and the fetus. Similar early reactivity was observed in cattle (BILLINGHAM, 1957). Very weak tolerance to allogeneic skin grafts can be induced in rabbits inoculated as newborn, though in only 25% (BILLINGHAM and BRENT, 1959). The developing rabbit embryo is able to react in the last trimester of pregnancy, PORTER (1960) estimated that the period in which tolerance can be induced (adaptive period) ends at the 22nd day of rabbit fetal life. Tolerance to allogeneic skin grafts can be induced in mice 24 hours after birth, but not in all strain combinations and only by i.v. injection; i.p. inoculation is usually ineffective. The responsiveness of the chicken is similar (HASEK, 1956). Tolerance can be induced in dogs by exsanguinotransfusion performed 24 hours after birth with an amount of blood which represents double the volume of the amount of blood in the newborn animals. The percentage of white blood cells in the donated blood used for induction of tolerance should be increased by some method of stimulation, e.g. repeated bleeding (PUZA and GOMBOS, 1958). In sheep the same procedure has little effect (GROZDANOVIC et al., 1959). Few such experiments have been performed in humans. First, the danger of the graft-versus-host reaction if immunologically competent cells were used to induce tolerance is too great. Secondly, there is the danger of transferring unknown viruses (including oncogenic ones) if any type of material derived from human cells is induced.

The animals which show the longest period in which tolerance can be induced are probably ducks (7 days after hatching; SVOBODA, 1958) and rats (7—10 days; BILLINGHAM et al., 1960). Most promising in this respect, however, may be the oppossum and the kangaroo (SOLOMON, 1971).

Development of the immunological apparatus in various species can be studied by comparing how soon during embryogenesis and after birth immunological reactions can appear. A large number of experiments have been addressed to this question. Thus, experiments involving only three species will be briefly summarized: the mouse, since it is a classical immunogenetic animal; sheep, because they have been subjected to the most advanced studies and man.

Various mouse embryo tissues contain cells which are precursors of immunologically competent cells. Precursors of cells capable of cell-mediated immunity were detected by means of the graft-versus-host reaction. However, these precursor cells must mature in the intermediate host. In such experiments, cells from mouse-embryo organs at various stages of development are injected into compatible hosts, i.e. sublethally irradiated F_1 hybrids. After a certain interval, lymphoid tissue cells from the intermediate hosts are transferred into another group of sublethally irradiated F_1 hybrids. Death of the latter hosts indicates a graft-versus-host reaction and that precursors of cells capable of producing such a reaction were present in the original embryonic tissue. This test system has shown that liver and placenta from a 9-day-mouse-embryo, yolk sac from a 12-day embryo, upper trunk and thymus from the 11th and 15th days of gestation, lung from the 15th day of gestation, bone marrow and spleen at the end of gestation and intestine after birth contain such cells (TYAN, 1968). Immediately after birth these cells can be identified in liver, Peyer's patches, lung, bone marrow, lymph nodes, spleen, blood and thymus (TYAN and COLE, 1965; McGREGOR, 1968). The functional development of these precursor cells is thymus-dependent (TYAN, 1964). With an adaptation of this system, cells which are precursors of immunoglobulin-producing cells were also identified. Such precursor cells were found in the yolk sac of a 9-day embryo, in the placenta of a 10-day embryo, and in intestine and lung from 16- to 20-day embryos. At the end of pregnancy, precursors of immunoglobulin-producing cells were found in bone marrow, spleen and blood (TYAN *et al.*, 1967). Precursors of immunoglobulin-producing cells may be independent of thymus, but may depend on the influence of intestinal lymphoid tissue (Peyer's patches) (PEREY *et al.*, 1968).

Newborn mice reject allogeneic skin homografts as rapidly as adult mice (STEINMULLER, 1961). COHEN *et al.* (1963) showed the presence of immunocompetent cells in mouse thymus at birth. The spleen cells from 18-day mouse embryos are unable to react *in vitro* against allogeneic target cells, but spleen cells from 1-day-old mice do react (AUERBACH and GLOBERSON, 1966). However, a rapid increase in immune cells of spleen can be observed within the first 12 weeks of life (DALMASSO *et al.*, 1963). The antibody response in newborn mice is less pronounced than the cellular response. For example, MOULTON and STORER (1962) did not detect any allo-antibody until the age of 30 days, BORAHES and HILDEMAN (1965), until the age of 11 days. The difference was probably caused by the different dosages of antigen used for immunization, among other factors.

A very important experiment concerning the development of immunological reactions during embryogenesis was performed on sheep by SCHINKEL and FERGUSON (1953). Recipient embryos rejected skin grafts from the mother at 110—117 days of gestation. Later, SILVERSTEIN *et al.* (1964) showed that lamb fetuses could reject skin allografts as early as the 85th day of gestation but that skin allografts applied prior to this time not only failed to be rejected but could induce tolerance. It is remarkable that the histological picture and time of rejection of skin allografts by fetal lambs are practically identical to rejection by an adult sheep, the rejection time being between 7 and 10 days.

Fetal lambs immunized *in utero* during the first half of pregnancy can produce antibody (SILVERSTEIN *et al.*, 1963; SILVERSTEIN and KRANER, 1965). It should be noted that even at the beginning of this century, antibody formation in fetuses after *in utero* stimulation was described by KREIDL and MANDL (1904). Fetal lambs do not respond equally well to all antigens. The best antigenic stimulus in this respect seems to be bacteriophage X 174, because it can immunize at the earliest technically possible time (38 to 40 days of gestation). At the age of 66 days, the fetus responds to ferritin and at the age of 120 days, starts to form antibodies against egg ovalbumin. The gestation period of a sheep is 150 days. After birth, active antibody formation occurs against diphtheria toxin and *Salmonella typhosa* (SILVERSTEIN *et al.*, 1963).

FOWLER *et al.* (1960) studied the fate of skin grafts from blood donors in children treated with blood transfusions for hemorrhagic jaundice. When fresh blood was used, some degree of tolerance was detected. On the other hand, a prematurely born baby with an estimated gestational age of 32 weeks was able to reject its father's skin graft within 12 days. The formation of humoral antibodies must also begin very early in human embryonic life. Small lymphocytes appear at the 7th to 8th week of gestation (PLAYFAIR, 1963). Synthesis of IgM was detected a few days later — at 74 days (GITTLIN and BIASUCARI, 1969). IgG could be detected at 84 days, and IgA at 95 days. Experimental immunization cannot be performed, but natural transplacental immunization serves as a source of the type of data already known from other mammals. For example, antibodies against rubella virus can be produced by a 112-day fetus (BURNET, 1960). Similarly, a reaction against treponema can be detected in early human embryos (SILVERSTEIN and ZUCKERS, 1962). Under normal conditions, only IgG can pass from the mother to the fetus. Finding of IgM or IgA indicates active synthesis by the fetus. SEVER and BERENDES (1967) found elevated IgM in connection with rubella.

The problem of the mother-fetus relationship are complicated. For example, why does the mother not react against the normal transplantation antigens of the embryo, which are different from hers (the embryo is actually an allograft)? Why does the embryo not develop tolerance or immunity against the mother's normal transplantation antigens?

Several hypotheses have been offered to explain the mother's nonreactivity, none of which are fully satisfactory. The theory that the embryo is antigenically immature no longer holds and is mentioned only because it was proposed first. UPHOFF (1970) suggested a maternal modification of the embryonal antigenicity as a mechanism which aids in the survival of the fetus. This theory is interesting in connection with the example of antigenic modification and modulation (see p. 5). From the point of view of CEA, however, it is important not only to increase our knowledge of the development and modification of normal antigens during embryogenesis, but also to determine whether they are stage-specific (ANDERSON, 1971). The existence of such stage-specific antigens in various species, including man, is extremely likely. Specificity of antigens which are limited in their existence only to a certain period of time and to certain organs could play an important role in embryogenesis and organogenesis. What better, more specific and more natural markers could there be on the surface of the cells than membrane-associated antigens? We know that antibodies and immunocompetent cells, which have all of the tools to recognize and interact with such markers, occur very early in embryonic life. The existence of stage-specific antigens during normal embryonic development, antigens which can reappear after malignant transformation, could explain the uniqueness of tumor-specific antigens for a given type of tumor. Each oncogenic virus, for example, could derepress different stage *and* organ-or-tissue-specificity. To my knowledge, no one has yet studied stage specificity of embryos of warm-blooded animals. ROMANOVSKY (1960), however, reported the presence of various antigens at various stages of development of axolotl larvae (*Amblyostoma mexicana*).

The decreased reactivity of the mother during pregnancy has been experimentelly documented in several species and is probably caused by increased production of adrenocortical hormones. HESLOP *et al.* (1954) showed a significant prolongation of surviving skin allografts in rabbits. On the other hand, this effect was observed neither in mice (MEDAWAR and SPARROW, 1956) nor in cattle (BILLINGHAM and LAMPKIN, 1957). SCHLESINGER (1962) proved that the uterus is not an immunologically privileged site. Not only pregnancy, but mating with a sterile male can induce a certain degree of immunologic nonreactivity to normal transplantation antigens of the paternal strain (PREHN, 1960). On the other hand, it is not certain whether such decreased reactivity plays a useful role in the survival of the fetus, since active immunization with paternal and maternal antigens does not influence normal development of transplanted ova in rabbits (LAUMAN *et al.*, 1962). GOODLIN and HERZENBERG (1964) found that C 57 Bl/6 females mated with DBA/2 males produced hemagglutinins against paternal erythrocytes. Such immunity did not influence the fetus or the fertility of the female. This experiment provides additional proof that the mother is able to react immunologically against her own fetus. Such an observation contradicts the hypothesis that mother and fetus are separated by an anatomical barrier. In mammals with a hemochorial placenta (e.g. man) the amount of space in the placenta between the mother and fetal tissue is almost negligible. In rats, such a barrier can exist, at least to cells introduced from the mother into the fetuses. When a rat uterus containing embryos is irradiated (15-day embryos) with 200 rads, thus damaging the placental barrier, specific tolerance to the mother's transplantation antigens is induced in a large percentage of the offspring (LENGEROVA, 1957). Even under normal conditions, some tolerance to the mother's antigens exists in guinea pigs (BILLINGHAM *et al.*, 1956) indicating that in this species, the barrier is not very strong.

It has recently been demonstrated (BEER *et al.*, 1972; BEER and BILLINGHAM, 1973) that immunocompetent cells can pass through the placenta of some species and cause immunological damage to the histoincompatible embryos. More than half of the offspring of female Fischer rats mated with Fischer males developed runting syndrome if the hematopoietic apparatus of the pregnant mother was replaced (after immunosuppression with cyclophosphamide) with bone marrow from Lewis rats. Runting syndrome was also obtained when the pregnant Fischer rats were injected with lymphoid cells from Lewis rats presensitized against Fischer antigen. This reaction is dose-dependent; an increased number of immunocompetent cells can increase the incidence of runting syndrome to 91%. The antigens against which the transfer cells react must belong to the rat major Ag-B locus, otherwise the reaction is negligible. It seems that stimulated immune cells can pass through the placenta better than normal immune cells. It is also likely that allogeneic lymphocytes can survive for several weeks after transfer to normal, unsensitized pregnant females, regardless of their compatibility at the Ag-B locus with the host cells. Results similar to those obtained in the rats were obtained in mice, hamsters and rabbits. These findings are very important, as they indicate that the fetus can be damaged by the mother's immunologic reaction even when the structural integrity of the placenta has not been altered by irradiation or drugs. Moreover, active immunization of the mother can lead to runting syndrome, but only under certain conditions. The most important factors seem to be timing and dosage. Hyperimmunization can lead to production of protecting (blocking, enhancing) antibodies (HELLSTRÖM *et al.*, 1969) which prevent the runting syndrome from being detected.

In previous experiments in which no effect of the pregnant females' hyper-immunity on development of the embryos had been observed, the negative results may be the result of overwhelming the cellular immune system with blocking anti-bodies, or the method of detection. Most investigators were looking for a classical type of transplantation reaction which would be manifested by rejection of or immediate damage to the embryos. The runting syndrome, first described by BILLINGHAM does not develop for several weeks after birth.

Why does the fetus not respond either with tolerance or immunity against maternal antigens? Sometimes the fetus actually does develop tolerance. In addition to an anatomical barrier, an immunological barrier between the mother and the fetus can exist as well though more functional than structural. This possibility was shown by HELLSTRÖM *et al.* (1969). They used *in-vitro* methods to show that the mother has cytotoxic immune cells against fibroblasts of her own embryo(s). The serum of the mother contained blocking factors (enhancing antibodies), which were able to protect the embryo cells *in vitro* against the action of the mother's immune cells. This blocking function probably also operates during pregnancy *in vivo*. The possi-bility that enhancement is induced by multiparity was suggested earlier (KALISS and DAGG, 1964). The simultaneous presence of immune cells with cytotoxic activity and of antibodies with blocking activity very much resembles the enhancement in syngeneic systems in tumor immunology (BUBENIK and KOLDOVSKY, 1964; MÖLLER, 1964; cf. HELLSTRÖM, 1971).

In summary it can be said that a developing organism always expresses some cell membrane-associated antigens. Such antigenic expression increases in quantity and quality during development. It is probable that some of these antigens are present only for certain periods of time in certain organs and tissues, thus constituting stage-specific antigens. An immunological apparatus develops rapidly at the same time. Since the separation between mother and fetus is far from complete, one would expect immunological reactions between mother and fetus (immunity or tolerance). Certain immune reactions play a role in embryo- and organogenesis and in protecting the fetus from unwanted immune reactions of the mother. Abnormal reactions (like hemorrhagic) can occur, however, and cause immunologic damage to the embryo, though most embryos develop to maturity without such damage.

IV. Tumor-Specific Antigens

Tumor-specific antigens are detectable only in malignant tumors and not in adult tissue under normal conditions. Many such antigens have been found in experimental tumors. One can say that practically every experimental tumor which was examined carefully enough was shown to contain these antigens. In the rare cases when such antigens were not found, one can always say that the search was not thorough enough. The search for such antigens in human tumors in recent years has produced evidence that human tumors also contain such antigens.

Several types of tumor-specific antigens occur in experimental tumors. These antigens can be differentiated by methods of detection, cell localization, other biological properties and by significance for tumor growth. Generally speaking, these antigens can be divided into three groups (cf. KOLDOVSKY, 1970) and will be discussed in terms of their importance for tumor growth, from the aspect of clinical immunology.

The tumor-specific transplantation antigen (TSTA) is the most important because an immunologic response against this antigen can be detected very early (giving it prospective diagnostic value) and can influence tumor growth significantly, either by inhibiting tumor growth (resistance against tumor, prospective immunotherapy) or by promoting tumor growth (enhancement). Although transplantation immunity against tumors was observed a long time ago, in the early experiments most of the reaction was directed against normal transplantation antigens which are also present on the surface of the malignant cells. The development of inbred strains of animals by sibling mating (mainly in mice, which are highly antigenically homogeneous), led to the possibility to induce specific antitumor reaction exclusively. Within an inbred population, all animals are antigenically identical. When a tumor does appear within such a population, it first exhibits the same transplantation antigens as the normal tissues of such animals. When, however, the malignant tumor contains additional antigen(s) not present in the normal tissue, this positive antigenic change can be detected with relative ease by preimmunization and transplantation tests. Animals of an inbred population shown to be antigenically homogeneous by previous skin graft tests are immunized with a tumor which is indigenous in the given population. Subsequently, the immunized animals are injected with living cells from the same malignant tumor. If the tumor contains a new antigen (TSTA), the animal will not support tumor growth, and resistance to (no growth) or inhibition of tumor growth will be detected. The reaction is not absolute; the animals should be tested with a limited, known number of tumor cells. Usually this number represents only a few minimal doses of cells (a minimal dose of tumor cells is that dose which leads to the growth of tumors in 100% of the control animals). The control animals should be immunized with syngeneic normal tissue (to determine the antigenic homogeneity) and other control animals should be immunized with unrelated normal or malignant tissue (to monitor nonspecific stimulation). Similarly designed experiments were performed by LUMSDEN (1929) but solid evidence came from the experiments of GROSS (1943) on methylcholanthrene-induced tumors in mice. The most convincing evidence that such new antigens are tumor-specific and not a mutation of a normal transplantation antigen came from the experiments of KLEIN *et al.* (1960). They demonstrated that after surgical removal of the primary tumors mice could become resistant to transplantation of the same tumor, an example of a real autoimmune reaction.

TSTA were demonstrated in tumors induced by carcinogens: carcinogen-induced leukemia (GORER and AMOS, 1956), benzpyrene- (KOLDOVSKY, 1960), dibenzanthracene- (PREHN, 1960), urethane- (PREHN, 1962), and other carcinogen-induced mammary carcinomas (PREHN, 1962). The presence of TSTA in so-called spontaneous tumors (mostly mammary carcinomas) was for a long time doubted because many negative results were obtained with these tumors. One explanation is that natural immunological tolerance can exist against these tumors or that natural immunological tolerance can exist against their TSTA. In 1963, AXELRAD proposed the possibility of natural immunological tolerance against TSTA of some tumors. Later, it was demonstrated in a series of experiments by P. BLAIR and others (cf. WEISS, 1967) that tolerance plays an important role in the reactivity of mice against spontaneous mammary carcinoma in C 3 H mice. Briefly, mice of C 3 H origin, when nursed by virus-free forster mother (C 57 Bl) and thus free of milk-borne mammary virus infection, can relatively easily be made resistant against mammary tumor. Normal C 3 H mice under similar conditions have no detectable reaction against this tumor. It was shown recently (Symposium on mammary virus neoplasia, Cherry Hill 1971) that normal mice carrying the mammary tumor virus can react when hyperimmunized against mammary tumors. These findings are important for understanding the appearance of TSTA in tumors. Spontaneous carcinomas of the mammary gland are undoubtedly of virus origin. Following the original discovery of SJOGREN *et al.* (1961) that polyoma virus induces a new TSTA, it was found that practically all oncogenic viruses induce new TSTA (cf. SJOGREN, 1964). Thus it was difficult to understand why mammary carcinomas should not have this antigen.

One important difference exists between virus- and carcinogen-induced tumors: tumors induced by certain viruses contain common specific TSTA for all tumors induced by the same virus, while the tumors induced by chemical carcinogens have TSTA which are individually specific (SJOGREN, 1964).

As mentioned above, TSTA has been detected in most experimental tumors. Because no transplantation experiments can readily be performed, the presence of TSTA in humans cannot be studied directly. The most progress in this respect was achieved by means of *in-vitro* methods for studying cell-mediated immunity. It is most probable that immune cells react against target cells *in vitro* and destroy them because of the reaction against the same surface antigens which caused the transplantation reaction. The *in-vitro* reaction against normal transplantation antigens was known many years ago. MURPHY (1926) performed ingenious experiments in which he let pieces of tissue grow on the allantochorion of chicken embryos. Nearby he grafted a piece of spleen or lymph node. The immune tissue inhibited the growth of the normal tissue only when specific immune tissue in combination with antigenically incompatible target tissue was used. Later Lumsden (1931) observed a completely *in-vitro* reaction of immune cells against target cells. The immune cells were obtained *in vivo* from a preimmunized donor. More recently Rosenau and Moon (1965) showed that immune cells can destroy target cells *in vitro* when there is a difference at the H-2 locus or only at the TSTA. Koldovsky (1965) and Koldovsky and Axler (1970) showed that the anti-H-2 antigen reaction can be performed *in vitro*, including primary stimulation. The same was demonstrated *in vitro* for the heterologous reaction (rat × mouse) by Winocour and Sachs (1965).

Hellstrom and Sjogren (1965) developed a new technique for detecting and measuring anticellular immunity mediated by immune cells *in vitro*. This technique, called colony inhibition, consists of plating immune cells on top of a small quantity of target cells. The colonies of target cells are counted one week later and the results are compared with those obtained from colonies which grow from target cells treated with corresponding nonimmune cells. Another technique based on a similar principle was also developed in which target and immune cells are plated in small wells of microplates (Tagasuki and Klein, 1971). In cases of pronounced immunity, the destruction of target cells by immunocompetent cells *in vitro* can be determined by the ^{51}Cr-release technique (Brunner, 1971). All of these techniques probably really measure the reaction against cell membrane-associated (transplantation) antigens.

It has been shown in many laboratories, though originally and mainly by the Hellströms (Hellström *et al.*, 1972), that cancer patients often have in their peripheral blood cytotoxic immune cells against their own tumor cells grown *in vitro*. The wide cross-reactivity observed in human tumors is interesting to note. Practically all tumors of the same type exhibit cross-reacting antigenicity. For example, lymphocytes from a patient with neuroblastoma will react *in vitro* not only with his own neuroblastoma cells but also with any other neuroblastoma derived from different patients. The lymphocytes will not react against normal cells (skin fibroblasts) of autologous or allogeneic origin, nor will they react against tumor cells of different origin (e.g. lung carcinoma). This observation indicates that a common tumor-specific antigen exists in human tumors of the same histogenetic origin. If one can extrapolate from experiences in animals, it could mean that all tumors of the same type are induced by the same virus. However, an oncogenic virus responsible for human malignant tumors has not yet been isolated, despite prodigious efforts. Another possible explanation for this reaction is that antigens other than tumor-specific antigens are responsible for this reaction. Cross-reactivity may be caused by already-established concomitant infection, for example by mycoplasmas. A high proportion of human cell lines are actually contaminated by mycoplasmas and a large percentage of the population has antibodies (most likely, immune cells as well) against mycoplasma. Thus some of the reactions of cells and sera from tumor patients observed against tumor cells *in vitro*, may be directed against such antigens. However, this remark should be taken mainly as a warning of the many dangers which confront anyone who is studying antitumor immunity and who gets positive results. Two other types of antigens which are more likely to be responsible for such cross-reactions were recently discussed at a Symposium of Applied Tumor Immunology (1972).

One such antigen can be organ- or tissue-specific. After malignant transformation, cells probably retain most of their normal surface antigens including the organ- or tissue-specific ones. Persistence of organ-specific antigens has already been proved (NAIRN *et al.* 1966 KOLDOVSKY *et al.* 1972). Every organ or tissue may contain a specificantigen and that every tumor originating from that organ or tissue can have an organ- or tissue-specific antigen corresponding to the organ of origin. The other antigen, the so-called carcinoembryonic antigen CEA, soon to be the main topic of discussion, may result from derepression of some embryonic function.

In addition to cytotoxic cells (peripheral immune lymphocytes) in the serum of tumor patients, blocking factor (enhancing antibodies?) may be already bound to the tumor tissue *in situ* (DE WITT, 1972).

The second antigen to be discussed is the neoantigen or complement-fixing (CF) antigen which occurs in tumors induced by oncogenic viruses. This antigen can be detected by complement fixation, immunofluorescence and agaroprecipitation. In tumors induced in hamsters by adenoviruses HUEBNER *et al.* (1962) were unable to recover the virus but detected specific complement-fixing (CF) antibodies against tumor extract in the tumor-bearing animals. These antibodies are specific for a given type of adenovirus (HUEBNER *et al.*, 1963). CF antigen was detected in SV_{40}-induced tumors, which were studied extensively by GILDEN *et al.* (1965). In the case of DNA virus-induced tumors, CF antigen is a cellular component genetically controlled by the viral genome (cf. DEFENDI, 1971). The RNA virus-induced tumors also contain CF antigen, and sera form tumor-bearing hamsters (which are almost always of the nonproducing type) will react in the CF reaction with tumor extracts from Rous tumors of various origins. These sera will also react with tissue-culture cells infected with viruses which belong to the avian leukosis complex (HUEBNER, 1964). In contrast to DNA virus-induced tumors, however, CF antigen is an internal viral component (BAUER and SCHAFER, 1965).

The most obscure group of tumor-specific antigens were first described many years ago. These antigens were found by means of heterologous sera produced in animals (most often in rabbits) against various human or experimental tumors and absorbed with normal tissue. Such sera should specifically react only with the tumor tissue (or with extracts of tumor tissue). Various reactions were used for this purpose, most often the complement-fixation reaction and precipitation in agar. In the beginning, incorrect observations were made because the antigens detected were not tumor-specific. The antiserum detected the difference in blood-group antigens in the tumor tissue and in the tissue used as control and for absorption. Another incorrectly interpreted antigen was necroantigen. Bacterial antigens, organ-specific antigens, etc. can also easily be mistaken for tumor-specific antigens (DAY, 1966). The main problem, still not sufficiently solved for human tumors, is to find suitable control tissue for performing absorption and negative control reactions. After his initial studies in tumor immunology, WITEBSKY (1932) returned to this problem (1956) and again found differences between normal and malignant tissue even when he used more sensitive serological methods. With these methods, however, the difference was only quantitative. The same observations have often been made since that time. This question will be discussed in more detail in connection with CEA. When the system can detect antigen at the level of 10 mg/100 ml, under conditions in which normal tissue contains only 1 mg/100 ml, and tumor tissue several tens of mg, the reaction appears very specific and can, in fact, have great diagnostic value. In a strict immunological sense, however, this antigen is not tumor-specific. For example, quantitative antigenic differences between normal and malignant tissue have been found only by DULANEY *et al.* (1949), WISSLER *et al.* (1956), and HIRAMOTO and NUNGESTER (1958).

One objection to the use of heterologous sera of detecting tumor-specific antigen is that it is not sensitive enough. As will be seen later, very low levels of carcino-embryonic antigen (2 ng/ml), i.e. levels found in any healthy individual, can be detected by radioimmunoassay. Individual differences, particularly in human tumors, are difficult to compensate for when using heterologous sera. A serum produced against a single human tumor can be specific for this tumor and even cross react with some other tumor, which may accidently contain the same (and rare) normal antigen(s). It is possible to absorb such serum with normal human tissue pooled from many donors, but such absorption has two dangers, 1) it may absorb too much and 2) there may be no guarantee that a particular pool will contain all of the normal minor antigens. For example, BJORKLUND (1969) performed extensive adsorption studies using pooled tissue from ten healthy donors. This serum showed that the tumor-specific antigen was only three times more concentrated in the tumor than in the corresponding normal tissue.

These antigens may have diagnostic value if significantly high quantitative differences can regularly be detected for certain tumors. Such a system, however, is as yet undetected; if tumor immunology has a bad name, this group of antigens is probably responsible for it.

V. Carcinoembryonic Antigens

The name of this antigen is in itself a definition. It is an antigen whose occurrence is limited to normal embryonic tissue and, in adult organisms, to malignant tumors. CEA are divided into three major groups: 1) antigens expressed on the cell surface (cell membrane-associated CEA, transplantation CEA); 2) alpha globulins (alpha fetoprotein); and 3) CEA of the digestive tract.

1. Cell-Surface CEA

Almost from the beginning of experimental tumor immunology, as mentioned previously, it was observed that immunization against tumor grafts with embryonic tissue is more effective than immunization with corresponding normal adult tissue. This difference, however, can be caused by many factors which have nothing to do with CEA. In addition, many of the early experiments were not intended to demonstrate this difference.

In recent years, the possibility of the existence of CEA has attracted more attention and the evidence for the existence of the cell membrane-associated carcinoembryonic antigen is growing. HOUGHTON (1962) observed that rabbit antimouse erythrocyte serum agglutinated ascites tumor cells. FURUSAWA *et al.* (1965) concluded that mouse erythrocytes and Ehrlich ascites tumor cells contain a common antigen, agglutinogen, which is located on the inner surface of the erythrocyte membrane but on the outer surface of the tumor cell. In other words, the outer surface of the tumor cell and the inner surface of the erythrocyte have an antigen in common. FURUSAWA *et al.* (1966) then extended their study to include a comparison with embryonic erythrocytes. They found that erythrocytes from adult animals have different antigens expressed on their surface than do 14-day mouse embryonic erythrocytes. More important, in contrast to erythrocytes from adult mice, the embryonic erythrocytes share some surface antigens with Ehrlich ascites tumor cells.

SEDALLIAN and JACOB (1967) prepared sera in guinea pigs and rabbits against mouse embryo cells. In the absence of complement, these sera agglutinated Ehrlich ascites tumor cells at dilutions as high as 1:512. When complement was added, cytotoxic reactivity was detectable, and there was great variation in the properties of the various serum samples. The sera could be divided in three groups: 1) sera with agglutinating activity and no detectable cytotoxic activity; 2) sera with weak cytotoxic activity against tumor cells; and 3) sera strongly cytotoxic (in high titer) and even exhibiting cytolysis. The third type of serum was obtained more often when the vaccine was produced from embryos younger than 12 days. When embryos over 15 days were used, no cytotoxic antibodies could be elicited. Serum of the third type when applied to mice in which Ehrlich ascites tumors were already growing, inhibited growth of the tumors. Sera of the first two types shortened the survival time of tumor-bearing mice (enhancement?).

Some human sera are cytotoxic for several human cell lines *in vitro* (LANDY *et al.*, 1961; GINSBURG, 1961; SOUTHAM, 1965). This toxic factor can be absorbed by tumor, placental and lymphatic tissue. SAXEN and PENTTINEN (1961) showed that 9% of all fresh human sera caused clumping of HeLa cells. This effect was observed only with fresh sera and could be abolished by absorption with HeLa cells. It was observed in 40% of sera from pregnant women and in 26% of sera from cancer patients (SAXEN and PENTTINEN, 1962). Attempts to separate the agglutinating and cytotoxic factors were unsuccessful. TAL *et al.* (1964) found that 90% of sera from cancer patients (120 cases) agglutinated HeLa cells, 16% of sera from patients with chronic non-neoplastic diseases (51 cases) and 13% of sera from normal persons (237 individuals). All 12 sera from the pregnant women were positive. Agglutination was also obtained with seven out of eight other tumor cell lines but not with cell lines derived from normal organs, e.g. liver or kidney. The agglutinating factor can be absorbed from the serum by many human and animal tumors and by human placenta. Human liver and kidney do not have such absorption capacity. The activity is in the beta-globulin fraction of the serum. The mechanism of agglutination is unknown. TAL suggested that this agglutination is caused by changes in the surface charge of the cells or in the level of seromucus in the serum. Later she found (TAL, 1965) that the agglutinating factor can be absorbed by cytolipin H, but not by similar glycosphingolipids. The agglutination can be inhibited by lactose but not by other disaccharides. The cell-surface receptor in this agglutination reaction is probably identical to cytolipin H.

BUTTLE *et al.* (1962, 1964) and BUTTLE and TRYAN (1967) used human tumor lines adapted for growth in cortisone-treated rats (TOOLAN, 1951, 1955). TOOLAN (1957) showed that these tumor-bearing rats developed immunity against such tumors. BUTTLE found that serum from cortisone-treated rats bearing human tumors prevented tumor growth in rats freshly treated with cortisone (1960).

In later experiments BUTTLE *et al.* (1962) compared the immunogenicity of various materials on the basis of their abilities to prevent growth of such tumor lines in cortisone-treated rats. They found that immunization against certain tumors with identical tumor (e.g. HSI against HSl) was most effective. However, soon after removal from patients, all rapidly growing sarcomas showed equally high immunogenic activity.

The antigen is very labile; it is destroyed by freezing and thawing and by prolonged storage. BUTTLE *et al.* (1964) compared tumors of various histological types and found differences among these tumors. Their results, along with similar results obtained with various normal embryonic and adult tissues are summarized in Table 1.

When sera from pregnant women were mixed with rat-adapted human tumor cells and injected into rats just treated with cortisone, 2 out of 50 sera inhibited tumor growth. Five out of seven sera from women with repeated abortions exhibited tumor growth-inhibiting activity. In additional experiments with rat tumors (e.g. Walker tumor), the rats were preimmunized with adult and embryonic rat tissue. The results however were less uniform and positive results were obtained only in isolated cases.

In mice (presumably randomly bred) immunized with mouse embryonic liver positive results were obtained when iron-dextran induced tumors were used as a target and negative with Crocker sarcoma. BUTTLE and TRYAN (1967) repeated these model animal experiments in various inbred strains of mice. The growth of twenty tumors induced by methylcholanthrene in BALB/c and C 57 Bl/6 mice was not influenced by preimmunization with embryonic tissue derived from the same inbred strains of mice. PREHN's experiments with methylcholanthrene-induced tumors and cross-reactivity with embryonic tissue were mentioned previously.

Table 1. Influence of immunization of rats with various human tissues (malignant and normal) on growth of rat adapted human tumor line

Human tissue used for immunization	Growth inhibition of human tumor adapted for rat (%)
Carcinoma of the breast	None
Fibrosarcoma	46
Carcinoma of the bronchus	50
Carcinoma of the liver	60
Carcinoma of the rectum	82
Melanotic sarcoma (H)	91
Synovial sarcoma	95
Chondroma	97
Melanotic sarcoma (M)	100
Adult serum	None
Adult spleen	None
Adult muscle	37
Placenta	74
Fetal muscle	79
Fetal spleen	96

BROWN (1970) showed that lymph-node cells from multiparous mice inhibited colony formation of methylcholanthrene-induced tumors of syngeneic origin grown *in vitro*. No such effect was observed against normal adult fibroblasts of the same origin.

More conclusive data were obtained from studies of virus-induced tumors in animals. PEARSON and FREEMAN (1968) compared the antigenicity of a polyoma-transformed hamster cell line (PTF) with that of a so-called spontaneous hamster tumor line (ITF), both originating from the same inbred strain of hamsters. They used rabbit antisera to test the cytotoxic reaction and the transplantation test on these tumor cell lines. An antigen present in PTF cells and detectable by the rejection reaction and by the cytotoxic test, was not present in the ITF cells. This new antigen is probably a polyoma virus-associated cellular antigen. They demonstrated that this antigen is also a component of a normal embryo cell from 12- to 14-day embryos. This antigen was not detectable either in spleen cells from adult animals or in mouse polyoma virus-transformed cells. Spleen cells from hamsters immunized with hamster embryo cells were cytotoxic *in vitro* for PTF cells. TEVETHIA and RAPP (1965), on the other hand, did not succeed in producing immunity against SV_{40}-TSTA with normal embryonic hamster fibroblasts. When sera from pregnant hamsters were tested against SV_{40}-transformed cells, embryonic cells and cells derived from adult animals by indirect membrane immunofluorescence, a cross-reacting antigen shared by SV_{40}-transformed cells and embryonic cells (RAPP and DUFF, 1970) was detected.

COGGIN et al. (1970, 1971, 1972) showed that SV_{40}-induced hamster tumor cells crossreact with hamster embryos not more than 14 days old. The hamsters were immunized with irradiated embryonic tissue and later were grafted with diffusion (semi-permeable) chambers containing tumor cells. In immunized animals was the growth of these tumor cells inhibited in comparison with cells growing in chambers placed in control hamsters. The fact that nonirradiated embryo cells (which can repopulate and mature) and older embryos did not cause this effect indicate the transient character of a given antigen in embryonic tissue. Surprisingly positive results were obtained with embryonal tissue from other species, including man.

In our experiments (KOLDOVSKY et al., 1972) we have detected an antigen cross-reacting with unfertilized mouse eggs and SV_{40}-transformed mouse cells. This antigen can be detected by cytotoxic (lytic) reaction caused by guinea pig anti-mouse-egg sera. The presence of this antigen seems to be limited to the stage of first cell division. This antigen was not detectable in SV_{40}-transformed cells from other species. Absorption experiments with cells transformed by guinea pig anti-mouse-egg, anti-mouse-SV_{40} and anti-mouse-spleen sera indicated presence of two antigens in SV_{40}-transformed cells, one crossreacting with mouse eggs (probably coded by virus-derepressed cellular genome) and one responsible for crossreaction of SV_{40}-transformed cells of various species (probably coded directly by viral genome).

TING (1968) was not able to induce any detectable transplantation resistance against polyoma-induced tumor cells by preimmunization with syngeneic embryonic tissue. He used nonirradiated embryonic tissue and two strains of mice, C 3 Hf/HeN and C 57 Bl/Ka. Similar negative results were reported by DEFENDI in the discussion following PREHN's paper (PREHN, 1967; in Crossreacting Antigens). BLAIR (1970) also obtained negative results with mammary tumors induced by mammary tumor virus when the mice were preimmunized with mouse (syngeneic) embryonic tissue.

HELLSTRÖM et al. (1970) described a transplantation-type antigen in human colonic carcinomas. This cross-reacts with fetal gut epithelium in cytotoxic tests in vitro. In the colony-inhibition test, they found that lymphocytes from the peripheral blood of patients with adenocarcinomas of the colon reacted positively with cells derived from colonic carcinomas and from fetal intestinal and liver epithelial cells. No colony inhibition was exhibited by the same lymphocytes against cells derived from adult colonic mucosa or fetal kidney. Control lymphocytes obtained from persons without cancer or with another type of cancer did not inhibit in-vitro growth of cells derived from intestinal adenocarcinomas or fetal intenstine. It was later shown (HOLLINGSHEAD et al., 1970) that this antigen is probably different from the antigen described as cross-reacting between tumors of the digestive tract and embryonic intestinal tissue (GOLD and FREEMAN, 1965). The HELLSTRÖMS also reported that immune cells derived from pregnant women exhibited cytotoxic activity against such tumors. It is important to note here HELLSTRÖM's finding (1970) that pregnant women have cytotoxic cells against cells derived from their own embryos in their peripheral blood, but they have the blocking factor as well. An interesting statistical fact is that the incidence of carcinomas of the colon is less frequent in multiparous women than in catholic nuns (FRAUMENI et al., 1969).

With basically the same technique, we confirmed HELLSTRÖM's results (KOLDOVSKY and WEINSTEIN, 1972). By immunization and extensive absorption, we prepared heterologous guinea-pig antisera against cells derived from human colonic carcinoma and against cells derived from human embryo organs (lung, intestine, skin, brain). Such sera showed not only cross-reactivity between both types of tissues — human colonic carcinoma and human embryo intestine — but also the possibility of full cross-absorption. In other words, cells derived from human embryo intestine absorbed the specific cytotoxic activity of antiserum against colonic carcinoma cells when tested again on colonic carcinoma cells (Table 2). These absorption experiments

Table 2. Activity of guinea-pig Antisera against human embryo and tumor cells

Cells	Antisera					
	non-absorbed		absorbed with normal tissues		absorbed with embryo or tumor tissue	
	Anti BTl 3	Anti El	Anti BTl 3	Anti El	Anti BTl 3	Anti El
Embryo intestine[b]	256[c]	256	16	16	<2	<2
Embryo lung[b]	256	256	<2	<2	<2	<2
BTB[a]	512	256	32	16	<2	<2
CB[d]	256	512	<2	<2	<2	<2
CAZ[a]	n.t.	n.t.	16	8	n.t.	n.t.
CA 4[a]	n.t.	n.t.	16	8	n.t.	n.t.

n.t. = not tested.
[a] Cell lines derived from adenocarcinoma colon.
[b] Cell lines derived from intestine of a 3-month-old embryo.
[c] Titer of cytotoxic antibodies.
[d] Skin-derived cells from patient with tumor BTl 3.

indicate how extensive is the degree of cross-reactivity between human malignant and normal human embryonic intestinal cells. There was no evidence for cross-reactivity against cells derived from lung or skin cells from the same embryos.

The experiments described above, do not confirm or exclude that additional specificity exists in human tumors or that human embryonic organs (tissues) have real embryonic stage-(tissue)-specific antigens not shared with tumors.

This CEA is certainly associated with the cell membrane but is not identical with TSTA, as we have shown for CEA and TSTA of SV_{40}-induced mouse tumors (KOLDOVSKY, 1972). Although the experiments described above do not indicate that this antigen is of the transplantation type (no transplantation reaction is induced by active immunization), one should not exclude the possibility that it may play some role in tumor growth *in vivo*.

BALDWIN *et al.* (1972) showed that hepatomas induced in Wistar rats by dimethylaminoazobenzene (DAB) (1955) and sarcomas induced by methylcholanthrene (1967) contain individual TSTA.

This CEA, which is detectable by membrane fluorescence and by the cytotoxic reaction using sera from multiparous rats, is a CEA which is probably different from the TSTA: 1) TSTA is tumor-specific in the experimental system used: this CEA is common to all tumors tested; 2) TSTA elicits detectable transplantation reaction but this CEA does not; 3) the serum from multiparous rats blocks the cytotoxic action of lymph node cells from multiparous rats, but does not block the action of cells from rats immune to TSTA.

Another possible explanation of this discrepancy was recently pointed out by KLEIN (1973). It is likely that not all membrane associated antigens can induce transplantation reaction. In other words there are differences in biological properties of antigens detectable by transplantation resistance (as in animal-tumor TSTA) and antigens detectable by *in-vitro* cell-mediated cytotoxicity (as in human malignant tumors). Sera from multiparous rats produce positive membrane fluorescence with these tumor cells. These sera were also cytotoxic *in vitro* for all tumor cells tested thus far. Lymph-node cells from multiparous rats were also cytotoxic. These results indicate that all tumors studied have this CEA in common. On the other hand, immunization of rats with living or heavily irradiated embryonic tissue did not influence the growth of subsequently grafted sarcomas or hepatomas.

2. Alpha Fetoprotein

As early as 1944, PEDERSON described in fetal bovine serum a protein — alpha globulin — which was not detectable in adult bovine serum. BERGSTRAND and CZAR (1956) later found a similar protein in fetal serum. This so-called alpha fetoprotein (AFP) is synthesized by the liver (GITLIN and BOESMAN, 1967; LINDER and SEPALA, 1968) and is a major serum protein of the early fetus, second in quantity only to albumin (GITLIN and BOESMAN, 1966). Twelve different species of mammals produce embryo-specific proteins which disappear shortly before or after birth (GITLIN and BOESMAN, 1967). TATARINOV (1966) demonstrated that during normal embryonic development, the level of AFP in humans gradually decreases; the level present at birth is less than 2% of that present at the third embryonic month, which is considered 100%. TATARINOV (1964) also showed that this antigen is present in patients with hepatocellular carcinoma. It was later shown that several human fetus-specific proteins exist (TATARINOV, 1968; VIERUCCI *et al.*, 1968). ABELEV (1963) reported the occurrence of embryo-specific alpha globulin in sera of mice with primary hepatomas (ABELEV, 1963; ABELEV *et al.*, 1963).

This fetal antigen (alphafetuin) is to a certain extent species-specific — at least human AFP is not homologous with bovine fetuin (KITHIER *et al.*, 1968). The AFP of mice (ABELEV *et al.*, 1963) and monkeys (HULL *et al.*, 1969) is produced by the tumor cells themselves. In humans, it is probably released from the tumor directly into the blood stream: after surgical removal of the tumor by partial hepatectomy, AFP was often no longer detectable in the blood serum (MORKOV and SOKOLOV, 1970). ENGELGARDT *et al.* (1971) and GUSIEV *et al.* (1971) used immunofluorescence and found AFP in only a limited number of tumor cells obtained from patients with hepatocellular carcinomas. These patients had a positive fetoprotein level in serum. These AFP positive cells usually form three-dimensional foci and are often located near blood vessels and capillaries. Hematoxylin-eosin staining did not show any morphological differences between AFP-negative and AFP-positive tumor cells.

Immunofluorescence seems to be less sensitive for AFP detection than is agaro-precipitation. Using immunofluorescence, NISHISKA *et al.* (1972) found AFP in

tumor cells from 9 out of 10 patients with primary hepatocellular carcinoma. In
these experiments, however, immunofluorescence was more sensitive than radial
immunodiffusion or the Ouchterlony technique. AFP was found to be localized in
the cytoplasm, the cytoplasmic membrane and the perinuclear zone. The number
of positive cells represented one fifth or less of all tumor cells studied. AFP was
sometimes observed in the cytoplasm of Kupffer's cells but was absent from connec-
tive tissue, bile ducts and normal liver cells.

The degree of specificity of this antigen for primary hepatoma is an important
question. TATARINOV (1964) suggested its possible usefulness as a diagnostic tool
at the time of its discovery. Specificity in this type of antigen is always very dependent
on the sensitivity of the test employed, i.e., a more sensitive test will detect lower
levels of the antigen in more and more cases, and thus its specificity will slowly
"disappear". Extremely low levels of some of the antigens common to tumor and
embryonic tissue can be found in almost every person. A certain level, however,
could be considered normal, and above this level, the amount detectable could be
considered specific, i.e., of diagnostic (prognostic) value. The CEA illustrate this
situation clearly. For example, FOLI et al. (1969) used the immunodiffusion technique
to determine the presence of AFP in sera from 62 patients, the majority of them
had non-neoplastic liver diseases (cirrhosis, chronic hepatitis, viral hepatitis) and
found all sera to be negative for AFP. Sera from 14 out of 35 patients with hepatocellular carcinoma were positive. MASOPUST et al. (1968) used immunodiffusion,
immunoelectrophoresis and quantitative immunoelectrophoresis to study sera from
248 patients (adults and children) with tumors and 484 patients with non-tumor
diseases. In only 6 out of 248 patients with neoplastic diseases (2.4%) was the
reaction positive. The positive cases included 2 malignant teratoma and 4 hepatocellular carcinoma. Among the group with non-neoplastic diseases, AFP was detected
only in children under 12 years of age with hepatopathies. In the positive cases, the
level varied from 6—90 mg/ml of serum. Similarly, URIEL (1967) described AFP in
sera of patients with hepatocellular carcinoma and ABELEV (1967) in some patients
with hepatocellular and mixed liver carcinoma, and in patients with testicular
teratoma. The radioimmunoassay is far more sensitive for detecting AFP than
immunodiffusion, immunoelectrophoresis or immunofluorescence. ABELEV et al.
(1971) used autoradiography and aggregate hemagglutination and found not only
a higher percentage of patients with hepatocellular carcinoma and teratomas who
reacted positively but also detected AFP in sera from pregnant women and patients
with hepatitis. A high incidence of positive sera from patients with hepatomas was
reported by PURVES and PERSOHN (1969, 1970), and TATATINOV (1964) also found
positive sera from pregnant women and patients with hepatitis. RUOSLAHTI and
SEPPÄLÄ (1971) refined the radioimmunoassay so that as little as 250 pg/ml of AFP
can be detected, making the method at least 20,000 times more sensitive than the
immunodiffusion method. AFP can be detected by this method in almost every
person; the level varies primarily around 10 ng/ml and very rarely exceeds 20 mg/ml.
But even using a less sensitive method, "sandwich" counter immunoelectrophoresis,
which can detect microgram amounts, SMITH (1971a) showed that AFP is detectable
in sera from patients with viral hepatitis and in sera from pregnant women during the
second and third trimesters. Using the same technique, SMITH (1971b) noticed that
AFP can be detected transiently in the sera of adults during the course of viral

hepatitis associated with the Australia antigen but not with acute viral hepatitis unassociated with this antigen. Even here the sensitivity of the technique seems to be important, since RUOSLAHTI and SEPPÄLÄ (1972) detect AFP in both types of hepatitis (Australia antigen negative and positive) by radioimmunoassay.

Recently, EDYNAK et al. (1972) described another fetoprotein associated with human carcinoma. This antigen was detected by agaroprecipitation. Saline extracts of various tumors were used as antigen (ABELEV et al., 1967). They had been prepared by high speed centrifugation, lyophilization of supernatant and reconstitution in small volumes of distilled water. In the beginning, serum of a patient with breast carcinoma was used for identification of this antigen. Later, it was found that 8 out of 1518 cancer patients have the precipitation antibodies. This antigen was called gamma fetoprotein because of its electrophoretic motility and presence in sera and tissues of normal fetus. It is present in 75% of a wide varieta of benign and malignant human tumors and 11% of the sera of cancer patients. It was also found in 2 non-neoplastic diseased tissues (out of 101, ELGORT et al., 1972); in both cases there was inflamed intestinal tissue. It was not present in any normal human adult tissue or serum. Fetal sera from pig, cat, dog and cow have this antigen; and mouse, rat and chicken fetal sera were negative. It was not found in any animal tumor. Gamma fetoprotein is serologically distinct from other known systems, including alpha fetoprotein and CEA of the digestive tract.

3. Carcinoembryonic Antigens of the Digestive Tract

In the early sixties, GOLD and FREEDMAN (1965) realized that the lack of adequate normal tissue for absorption and control reactions was the greatest hindrance to attempts to prepare specific heterologous antitumor antibodies. Furthermore, they felt that immunization of an animal (e.g. rabbit) just with human malignant tissue would lead to the production of too broad a spectrum of antibodies to the various antigenic components of such tissue. As a result there would be no assurance that the immunized animal is reacting against the tumor-specific antigen at all. To prepare specific antibodies just by absorption, i.e. by removing all unwanted antibodies and leaving the desired ones unharmed and in sufficient quantity is not a simple task. Thus, before they started their experiments, they established certain criteria:

1) Animals (rabbits) used for immunization should first be made immunologically nonreactive (tolerant) to normal human antigens. Under such conditions, immunization with tumor tissue can lead to a more specific response against the tumor antigens, i.e. the antitumor antiserum is more specific at the beginning of the absorption process (ZILBER et al., 1958; LEVI et al., 1959; KOLDOVSKY and SVOBODA, 1962).

2) Normal tissue from the donor of the malignant tissue should be used as a control. The normal tissue should correspond histologically to the malignant tissue.

3) A comparison should be made of the sensibility and reliability of immunological methods (tolerance, absorption) used to demonstrate the uniqueness of tumor antigenic constituents. In November, 1964, GOLD and FREEDMAN (1965) sent for publication their first paper on the antigenicity of tumors of the digestive tract. They selected this type of cancer because well-controlled, histologically corresponding normal tissue could be obtained with relative ease from the same patient. A

central cancerous portion of the tumor was used as the source of malignant material for immunization. Tissue more than 7 cm from the grossly visible edges of the tumor did not contain any (even microscopically) detectable malignant cells. Extracts were prepared from such normal and malignant tissues (pooled from patients and used for immunization, tolerance induction and absorption). From 12 hours after birth, rabbits were injected repeatedly for long periods with extracts from normal tissue and were later immunized with extracts of malignant tissues mixed with equal volumes of complete Freund's adjuvant. A control group of rabbits was immunized without being made tolerant. Antisera obtained were diluted 1:4 and absorbed with antigen in soluble form. The sera were tested by agaroprecipitation, immuno-electrophoresis and the hemagglutination reaction. Several antigens common to the colon and colonic carcinoma were detected. From the reactions obtained with the sera from tolerant rabbits, they concluded that tumor extracts contain additional antigens not detectable in normal colonic tissue. These antigens were detected by this antiserum in a number of individual colon carcinomas. The authors, however, carefully pointed out that it was not yet clear whether these additional antigens make the tumor tissue qualitatively or only quantitatively different from normal tissue. In a further study (GOLD and FREEDMAN, 1965b), they compared the antigenic composition of different adult normal, malignant and embryonic tissue, using the above described antiserum with the agaroprecipitation and precipitin inhibition reactions. A total of 322 human tissue samples were studied for their capacity to inhibit formation of the precipitin line between the antiserum and tumor extract. Precipitin inhibition was obtained with all 40 specimens of primary carcinoma of the digestive tract as well as from metastatic tumors of the same type. These results were confirmed by the direct precipitation reaction. All adult tissues — normal, diseased, nondigestive tract tumors — gave negative results in both tests. Negative results were also obtained with other tumors (e.g. ovarian carcinoma) metastasizing in the digestive tract. Precipitin inhibition was obtained with extracts of organs (gut, liver, pancreas) from human embryos between 2 and 8 months of gestation. Direct precipitation was obtained with the same organs from 2- to 6-month-old fetuses. This age difference in results with both reactions may reflect the greater sensitivity of the first reaction and the fact that as already mentioned for AFP, the amount of this CEA gradually decreases with the increasing age of the fetus.

When purified CEA of the digestive tract was prepared, GOLD (1967), using a modified bis-diazotized benzidine-hemagglutination method, followed the presence of anti-CEA antibodies in sera from 212 persons. No such activity was found in patients with metastatic cancers of the digestive tract. Positive reactions were observed in 70% of cases with digestive cancer without metastases, in a majority of sera from pregnant and postpartum women, and in two cases (5%) of noncancerous diseases of the digestive tract (both patients were treated by intestinal surgery and were over 60 years old). The sera of all other patients and healthy persons showed no anti-CEA activity.

Studies of the localization of CEA by immunofluorescence (GOLD et al., 1968) and by cytoagglutination (VON KLEIST and BURTIN, 1969) showed that CEA is closely associated with the cell membrane. Only electron microscopy combined with labeled antibodies could indicate where the antigen is localized. For this purpose, specific goat gamma globulin against purified CEA was prepared and labeled with ferritin. Using this serum and fresh, viable colonic cancer tissue, GOLD *et al.* (1970) detected CEA on the cell membrane but in the glycocalyx of the surface of the colonic cancer cell.

From the beginning of the studies on CEA, it was not clear how specific this antigen was for cancer of the digestive tract. McNEIT *et al.* (1969) found that specific antiserum prepared in rabbits against pooled fluid from seven ovarian cysts showed cross-reactivity in agaroprecipitation with CEA of the digestive tract. Other mucin-producing tumors such as carcinoma of lung or breast failed to show such cross-reactivity.

HAKKINEN *et al.* showed in a series of experiments (1966, 1967, 1968a, b, 1969) that gastric juice contains three distinct sulphoglycoprotein antigens: 1) a common surface (superficial) gastric sulphoglycoprotein antigen; 2) an intestinal sulpho-glycoprotein antigen not present in the stomach of healthy young persons, but which can be present in deep gastric glands of persons with certain pathological conditions and in nondiseased stomachs of old persons; 3) a fetal sulphoglycoprotein antigen, which is present during the fetal period in superficial cells of the digestive tract epithelium and occasionally reappears later in adult life. It is also a product of gastric cancer cells with secretory activity. In 3 out of 25 cases, cells producing this antigen were found in ulcerated stomachs. Such findings, however, may be indicative of a precancerous stage.

MARTIN and MARTIN (1970) immunized rabbits with extracts of colonic cancer and detected again two cancer-related antigens. These antigens could be demonstrated by agaroprecipitation in extracts from rectal adenocarcinomas, gastric cancer and fetal intestine, but not in extracts from noncancerous adult digestive tract. With the precipitin inhibition reaction, however, these antigens could be demonstrated in extracts from normal digestive tract mucosa, though in concentrations considerably lower than those in extracts from digestive tract tumors. Inhibition of the precipitin reaction usually requires 1.25—20 mg of antigen when extracts from malignant tissues are used: similar inhibition could be obtained only with 80—160 mg of extract of noncancerous tissue, and some noncancerous tissue failed completely to inhibit the precipitin reaction even at this concentration. It is interesting to note that cases of adenocarcinoma of the colon have a higher concentration of this antigen than adenocarcinomas of the stomach; a similar relation is present in corresponding normal tissue. BURTIN *et al.* (1970) prepared specific antisera against CEA and demon-strated its presence in two human digestive-tract carcinomas which were maintained *in vitro* for 8 and 7 years respectively. This important finding indicates not only the persistence of this type of antigen, but also that no maturation or histological change (selection) occurred during prolonged cultivation. The fact that malignant change can be accompanied by the loss of normal cell-surface antigens (H-LA, AB 0, H-2) was discussed previously. BURTIN *et al.* (1971) observed that the cell-membrane antigen of normal colonic mucosa was no longer detectable in carcinomas. The amount of this type of antigen was lower in cases of polyps of the colon in comparison with the level present in normal tissue. There seems to be an indirect correlation between loss of these antigens and reappearance of CEA in the digestive tract.

HOLLINSHEAD *et al.* (1970) prepared the soluble fraction of cell membranes obtained from carcinomas of the colon and rectum. There was a positive skin reaction to this preparation from 17 out of 19 patients. The same reaction was obtained using cell-membrane preparations from human embryonic digestive-tract cells. No reaction was obtained with membrane fractions prepared from normal cells. These skin-reactive antigens appeared to be closely related to CEA of the digestive tract. Later HOLLINSHEAD (1972), using polyacrylamide gel electrophoresis, found that CEA of the digestive tract discovered by GOLD, appears in a different region of the gel than the skin-reactive antigen.

4. As Yet Undefined Carcinoembryonic Antigens

There seem to be many CEA. Almost every time when a heterologous animal is immunized with fetal tissue and its serum tested, some new embryo-specificity is detected. Many of these embryo antigens then cross-react with malignant tumors. Do all tumors contain an antigen which has a counterpart in embryos at a certain stage and in certain tissue? Perhaps we should prepare a multivalent antiserum against all possible embryonic antigens and test it against all available tumors. When cross-reactivity is observed, one can attempt to determine which antigen is responsible for the cross-reaction.

STONEHILL and BENDICH (1970) prepared antisera in rabbits against extracts from whole mouse embryos of various periods of gestation. These sera were tested by agaroprecipitation before and after proper absorption with pooled normal mouse tissue. Basically, two antisera were compared — antiserum against 9-day mouse embryos and against 19-day mouse embryos — and then tested against the extract from various normal tissues and from 72 malignant mouse tumors. Antiserum against 19-day embryos reacted positively with all 72 malignant extracts but did not react with the extract of mouse L cells, or with many adult normal mouse tissue extracts. A positive reaction was also detected with extracts of skin, small intestine and regenerating liver. Serum against 9-day embryos reacted only with extracts of adult skin, 72 cancer extracts and embryonic and neonatal extracts.

KLAVINS et al. (1970) produced antibodies in rabbits against a lyophylized extract of a 6- to 7-week-old human fetus (from an ectopic pregnancy) mixed with Freund's adjuvant. The serum was again absorbed with normal human adult tissue and tested in the agaroprecipitation reaction. The serum reacted positively with all 6 extracts from various carcinomas (lung, breast, colon) and with extracts from normal adult skin. No reaction was detected with extracts of corresponding normal (lung) adult tissue.

YACHI et al. (1968) detected an antigen which exhibited partial cross-reactivity between embryonic tissue and tumor tissue extracts. From saline extracts of broncho-genic carcinoma, hepatome and colonic carcinoma, fractions soluble in 50% saturated ammonium sulphate were prepared and rabbits were immunized with these preparations. The sera obtained were absorbed with normal tissue extracts. Two tumor-specific antigens were detected from these antisera by agaroprecipitation. Both antigens were present in the carcinoma of the stomach, pancreas, liver and kidney. One of them showed a partial reaction with extracts from embryos. This antigen is probably not identical to AFP or CEA from the digestive tract.

These findings indicate that there are more CEA in the human tumors then just AFP and CEA of the digestive tract. The search for them is important both from a practical and a theoretical point of view.

VI. Properties of Carcinoembryonic Antigens

1. Transplantation CEA

As important as this antigen seems to be, little is known about it. It can be detected by its capacity of inducing resistance against the transplanted tumor. The same antigen is probably responsible for several *in-vitro* reactions: cytotoxic reaction by serum or immune cells, inhibition of *in-vivo* growth and *in-vitro* growth in diffusion chambers, colony inhibition, membrane fluorescence. When the reaction induced by this antigen is compared with reactions induced by other transplantation antigens, the transplantation CEA falls into the category of the so-called weak antigens. It is difficult to say whether this antigen exists in normal cells in some undetectable quantity or form (coated, covered, changed, deep inside the cell) or that it appears only after malignant transformation. It is probably coded for by the cell genome, even in virus-induced tumors which contain this antigen. Otherwise, since the same antigen is detectable during embryogenesis, it would be coded for in the embryonic cell by the same virus. The amount and the time of appearance of this CEA during embryogenesis may be important in determining whether the organism will be able to react against the antigen if it reappears in a tumor in the immunologically mature animal. Most antigens which are expressed during embryogenesis are recognized as self and are immunologically tolerated by the organism. This characteristic, however, may not be true for all antigens. First, the inducibility of tolerance seems to be limited in time. Not only can an antigen applied after birth (and in many cases during late embryogenesis) be too late to induce tolerance, but also an antigen applied too soon may not induce tolerance. For example, SIMMONSEN (1955) demonstrated that human erythrocytes induce tolerance only when injected in 14- to 19-day chicken embryos, but not before 14 days. Thus when CEA disappears early in embryogenesis, it must not induce tolerance. Also, tolerance need not last the whole life of the organism. For artificially induced tolerance, in fact, the opposite is more often the case. For example, a newborn rat injected with a certain antigen (human cells) exhibited tolerance when tested 2 months later but not when tested 3 months later. Although there is still no satisfactory answer to whether the continued presence of antigen is necessary to maintain tolerance, it is more likely that the presence is necessary. In some experimental systems it was found that the level of soluble protein (albumin) necessary to maintain tolerance should be 10 ng/ml. So when the amount of CEA decreases sharply after birth or disappears completely, tolerance can disappear as well. Also unknown is the optimal dose necessary to induce tolerance against various antigens during embryogenesis and the relationship of this dose to the real level of CEA, which can, during embryogenesis, be introduced into the immunological apparatus of the developing embryo. Also unknown is the form in which the antigen should be presented to the developing immunologic apparatus. The biophysical and biochemical properties of this antigen are also still unknown. A simple answer to this question does not exist even for normal transplantation antigens, which have been studied extensively in this respect.

2. Carcinoembryonic Antigens of the Liver Tumors — Alpha-Globulin

This antigen is not a subcellular component but a cellular product. A very low level of this antigen can be detected during the entire lifetime of the organism. The quantitative differences between normal adult organisms, embryos and certain types of cancer are, however, very large. The antigen is produced directly by the hepatoma cells. Alpha fetoprotein (AFP) has been detected in many species, each of which seems to have a different AFP. Only the human AFP will be discussed in this section. The concentration of AFP in human fetal serum is highest between 12—14 weeks of age, when it represents 10% of the total fetal protein. As birth approaches, it decreases rapidly. Human AFP cross-reacts with fetoprotein from rat, mouse (ABELEV, 1968) and baboon (PURVES, 1972). The AFP isolated from embryos and from hepatomas are antigenically and immunoelectrophoretically identical. RUOSLAHTI and SEPPÄLÄ (1971) purified AFP by electrofocusing and used the purified product to immunize sheep. The sheep antiserum was then used to prepare larger quantities of AFP by precipitation. The precipitate was dissolved and separated on a Sephadex G 200 column at pH 2.5. On electrofocusing, the AFP forms a single peak at pH 4.75. The small amounts of albumin and serum proteins accompanying AFP prepared in this way cause formation of antibodies after immunization; these must be absorbed with normal adult human serum. The immunochemically purified AFP reacts in immunodiffusion only with anti-AFP serum, and no reaction can be detected with antiserum against sheep gamma globulin. The purified AFP yields two electrophoretically distinct components on polyacrylamide gel electrophoresis. The molecular weight of the proteins in the electrophoretic bands was 140,000 and 70,000, respectively. The larger AFP was not detectable in fresh serum, but appeared after repeated freezing and thawing. The amino-acid composition of AFP is shown in Table 3. AFP contains 4.3% carbohydrate: 2.2% hexose, 1.2% hexosamine and 0.9% sialic acid. The molecular weight of human AFP differs from that of bovine AFP, which was determined by SPIRO (1960) to be 48,000. Analysis of the carbohydrates of both human and bovine AFP indicates that the two proteins are unrelated. RUOSLAHTI et al. (1971) compared the properties of AFP from human fetuses and from patients with hepatocellular cancer. They found that each protein is composed of a single polypeptide chain of molecular weight 70,000 and another of molecular weight 140,000. The amino-acid composition of fetal and cancerous AFP is very similar (see Table 4). When peptide maps of tryptic digests are compared, the localization of each peptide seems to be the same for both proteins. The carbohydrate composition of both proteins (total amount, relative amounts of various components) was also similar.

Localization of AFP can be followed by indirect immunofluorescence in primary hepatocellular carcinoma. This antigen can be found in cytoplasm, cytoplasmic membrane and perinuclear zone (GUSIEV et al., 1971). The fluorescence of tumor cells

Table 3. Amino acid composition of human α-fetoprotein, human albumin and bovine fetuin (Ruoslahti and Safállá, 1971)

Amino acid	AFP	Human albumin	Bovine fetuin
Asp	42.5	54.7	58.5
Thr	38.0	29.4	44.3
Ser	33.5	24.6	46.5
Glu	92.1	82.9	60.2
Pro	24.7	31.0	66.0
Gly	35.2	14.9	43.0
Ala	49.9	60.0	59.3
Cys	28.3	32.5	21.6
Val	31.3	46.0	71.0
Met	6.4	6.0	0
Ileu	57.9	63.5	47.8
Tyr	17.9	18.5	12.3
Phe	27.9	33.0	19.2
Lys	48.7	58.8	29.3
His	17.3	15.9	18.1
Arg	20.3	24.7	21.0
Try	undetermined	1	3.9

1. Brand, 1946; 2. Spiro and Spiro, 1962; 3. Moles of amino acid per 70,000 g glycoprotein; 4. moles of amino acid per 70,000 g peptide; 5. moles of amino acid recalculated per 67,000 g of peptide.

Table 4. Amino acid composition of human α-fetoproteins from fetuses and patients with a hepatocellular cancer (Ruoslahti and Sefállá, 1971)

Amino acid	Fetal fetoprotein	Hepatoma fetoprotein
Asp	42.5	44.0
Thr	38.0	34.4
Ser	33.5	39.2
Glu	92.1	101.0
Pro	24.7	23.3
Gly	35.2	34.9
Ala	49.9	50.4
Cys	28.3	31.7
Val	31.3	34.7
Met	6.4	7.3
Ileu	33.1	29.7
Leu	57.9	54.7
Tyr	17.9	17.1
Phe	27.9	28.6
Lys	48.7	45.8
His	17.3	16.3
Arg	20.3	21.3

Moles of amino acid per 70,000 g of glycoprotein.

appears in three forms: 1) diffuse, fine granular fluorescence of the cytoplasm; 2) the fluorescent line of the cytoplasmic membrane; 3) bright fluorescent line of the perinuclear zone. The first form is the most common. In many cases it is difficult to find any difference between the histological pictures of fluorescent positive and fluorescent negative tumor cells. Occasionally the fluorescent-positive cells show acidophilic granules in the cytoplasm.

It was proposed that embryo-specific proteins (embryo-specific alpha globulin) promote the growth of mammalian cells in tissue culture (MARZ et al., 1962).

3. Carcinoembryonic Antigens of the Digestive Tract (GOLD)

In preparing their antigenic material, GOLD and FREEDMAN (1965) used a simple extraction procedure: The homogenized tissue (pH 8.0) was first centrifuged and the sediment sonicated. Using ferritin-labeled antibodies, GOLD et al. (1970) showed that this CEA is localized in the glycocalyx of the surface of the cancer cell. This antigen is a seromucin. KRUPEY et al. (1968) studied the physicochemical properties of CEA of the digestive tract. Paper block electrophoresis of the perchloric acid extracts of normal and malignant tissue samples showed a number of components detectable by short-wave ultraviolet light. Although there were many similarities between the extracts of normal and malignant tissue, each specimen had its own distinctive pattern. Tumor antigenic material was always found at a certain position on the paper block (between 9 and 12 cm under the authors' conditions). When an eluate was prepared from this portion of the paper block, antigenic activity was found in the portion giving a spectrophotometric peak at 280 mμ.

The quantity of purified CEA varied with each tumor specimen: metastatic tissue, 0.001%, primary hepatoma, 0.005%, primary adenocarcinoma of the large bowel, 0.004%. The amino acids and their amounts in tumor samples are summarized in Table 5. Fucose was detected in tumor samples but not in the samples of normal tissue. Table 6 shows the carbohydrate composition. Ultracentrifugal analysis indicated a single peak and a sedimentation coefficient between 6.9 and 8.0 S. The primary adenocarcinomas and the metastatic tumors gave a single immunoelectrophoretic band with nonabsorbed rabbit anti-CEA antisera.

EGAN et al. (1972) showed that an established line of colonic adenocarcinoma cells produces CEA in vitro. In several determinations, more antigen was found in the medium in which the cells were grown than in the extract from the cells themselves. The antigen could be eluted from a Sephadex G 200 column in the same position as CEA extracted from tumor tissue. The amount of CEA increased with length of cultivation: a 7-day culture yielded 17 ng/ml, a 13-day culture 50 ng/ml, and a 29-day culture 300 ng/ml. Another line of colonic adenocarcinoma as well as eight other human cell lines from various sources were negative for CEA. Only one other human cell line, i.e., one established from an omental metastasis of a cervical carcinoma, was positive.

COLIGAN et al. (1972) compared CEA isolated from several tumors of the digestive tract, and found CEA of two molecular sizes, with sedimentation constants of 6.8 S and 10.1 S, respectively, the 6.8 S form being found more commonly. The content of the CEA from various tumors varies greatly. A comparison of the CEA prepared by GOLD and the authors showed that both products are immunologically identical. HAVERBACH and DYN (1972) reported that a clearer separation of antigen could be obtained when either ammonium sulphate or glycol, rather than perchloric acid, was used for extraction.

Table 5. Quantitative amino acid composition of the fractions possessing CEA activity
(KRUFEY *et al.*, 1968)

| Amino acid | Micromoles of amino acid per mg CEA | | | | | |
| | Specimen no. | | | | | |
	1	2	3	4	5	6
Asp	0.262	0.270	0.264	0.300	0.254	0.232
Thr	0.180	0.200	0.194	0.190	0.234	0.176
Ser	0.372	0.348	0.390	0.342	0.254	0.395
Glu	0.232	0.235	0.252	0.260	0.206	0.264
Pro	0.186	0.208	0.164	0.214	0.186	0.242
Gly	0.194	0.181	0.181	0.172	0.136	0.164
Ala	0.112	0.132	0.120	0.127	0.172	0.116
Ileu	0.040	0.052	0.044	0.046	0.024	0.038
Leu	0.016	0.020	0.018	0.016	0.017	0.016
Tyr	0.024	0.053	0.057	0.037	0.022	0.027
Phe	0.024	0.032	0.030	0.040	0.022	0.050
Lys	0.036	0.056	0.034	0.042	0.024	0.060
His	0.072	0.049	0.070	0.057	0.022	0.070
Arg	0.066	0.041	0.062	0.062	0.024	0.067
1/2 Cys	—	—	—	—	0.050	—

Table 6. Quantitative carbohydrate composition of the fractions possessing CEA activity
(KRUFEY *et al.*, 1968)

| Carbohydrate | Micromoles of carbohydrate per mg CEA | | | | |
| | Specimen no. | | | | |
	1	2	3	4	5
Fucose	0.834	0.965	0.902	1.060	0.623
Mannose	0.282	0.208	0.304	0.367	0.417
Galactose	1.000	0.924	0.867	1.104	0.562
Sialic acid	0.156	0.278	0.109	0.305	1.046

Sepharose 40 gel filtration revealed the presence of antigen in high and low molecular weight fractions, indicating the presence of several antigens or that the antigen forms complexes with itself. The molecular weight of the smaller molecule was about 170,000 to 200,000. Double-diffusion analysis of the preparative acrylamide gel fractions showed that the high molecular weight fraction has antigenic material with slow mobility and the low molecular weight fraction, has an antigenic component with fast mobility. This is a good indication that two CEA are present. Antigens extracted from bronchogenic carcinoma formed lines identical to antigens extracted from colonic carcinoma.

VII. Clinical Significance of Carcinoembryonic Antigens

1. Diagnostic and Prognostic Value

Theoretically, CEA of the transplantation type should elicit an immunological reaction very early in tumor development but there are as yet no adequate tests to detect the reaction. The only test available for detecting a reaction in the cancer patient — cell-mediated cytotoxic activity and blocking activity of the serum — is a complex test which cannot be performed routinely. Moreover, indications of the presence of the transplantation type of CEA exist only in adenocarcinoma of the digestive tract.

Promising results with other CEA indicate that they can be used diagnostically and prognostically.

In his first paper concerning detection of alpha fetoprotein in patients with liver tumors, TATARINOV (1964) proposed its usefulness in differential diagnosis of primary and metastatic liver tumors. ABELEV *et al.* (1967) compared the diagnostic value of finding AFP in patients with tumors (liver and other malignant tumors) and with noncancerous diseases of the liver. The sera from such patients were blind-tested and later correlated with results from clinical and histological examinations. AFP was determined by micro-agaroprecipitation and immunoelectrophoresis. Sera from a total of 308 patients were examined: 242 with cancer and 66 with noncancerous diseases. AFP was detected in 17 out of 28 patients with primary liver carcinoma and in 10 out of 47 patients with testicular tumors. All other sera, including sera from 67 patients with metastatic liver tumors, 66 nontumor liver diseases, were negative. It is interesting to note that teratoblastoma of the testis with features of embryonic carcinoma had the highest rate of positive reaction — 7 out of 17. MASOPUST *et al.* (1968) used double radial immunodiffusion in agar gel (OUCHTERLONY's plate method) and immunoelectrophoresis to search for AFP in sera from 248 patients with tumor diseases and 484 patients with different nontumor diseases. A positive reaction was detected only in two types of tumors: hepatocellular carcinoma (1 out of 3 cases) and malignant undifferentiated teratoma (4 out of 7). FOLI *et al.* (1969), using the immunodiffusion technique, found AFP in 14 out of 35 patients with hepatocellular carcinoma. The test was negative in all other patients. Analysis of the geographic localization of the patients with positive reactions showed that 5 out of 17 positives were British in origin, 5 out of 8 positives were West African and 4 out of 10 were from other regions. Thus the frequency of positive results in patients with hepatocellular carcinoma may be a regional difference. PURVES *et al.* (1970) followed the detection of AFP in patients with abnormal liver function, Bantu blood donors, neonates, Caucasian patients with primary cancer of the liver and male Bantu mine workers with primary liver carcinoma. No false positive AFP reaction appeared and the test was positive in 78% of primary liver cancer patients. No correlation of AFP with clinical data such as age, weight and survival time, was found. Neither was there any correlation of AFP with the weight of the tumor or of the liver. The nodule tumors produce the greatest amount of AFP. AFP production was low in the anaplastic (16 mg/100 ml), high in the poorly differentiated (32 mg/100 ml), and intermediate (25 mg/100 ml) in the well-differentiated tumors.

SMITH (1971) used a more sensitive method for detection of AFP (sandwich counter immunoelectrophoresis) which could detect concentrations of AFP of less than 100 ng/ml. He compared this technique with micro double-diffusion in agar and with the former found a higher incidence of positive sera in both tumor systems: the double-diffusion technique was positive for 5 out of 9 patients with primary hepatocellular carcinoma while with the sandwich counter immunoelectrophoresis technique, all 9 were positive. A similar difference was observed in patients with embryonic testicular carcinoma: 5 out of 20 patients were positive with the double-diffusion technique and 14 of the same 20 patients were positive with the more sensitive technique. With the more sensitive method, positive sera were found in 5 out of 15 cases of acute viral hepatitis, in 3 out of 11 pregnant women in the second trimester, in 8 out of 10 in the third trimester (0 out of 10 in the first trimester). All of these sera were negative in the double-diffusion technique. Sera from patients with other neoplasms with or without hepatic metastasis, fatty liver and cirrhosis, as well as from normal persons, were negative. TATARINOV (1964) detected a high level of AFP in sera from women who had just experienced spontaneous abortions. SMITH and O'NEILL (1971) made a comparative study of the appearance of AFP in various cases and found that AFP appears more frequently in teratocarcinoma (60%) than in embryonic-cell carcinoma (27%). In the patients with metastatic germinal cell tumors of the testis, detection of AFP seems to be related to the extent of the metastasis. Geographical differences have also been noted: 65% of the sera from persons from Hong Kong were positive, compared with 42% from the United States.

The experiments of HULL et al. (1969) are relevant to diagnosis. They induced hepatomas in monkeys and recorded the levels of AFP during cancerogenesis. AFP could be detected in monkeys (9 out of 14) before or at the time when hepatic nodules became palpable.

PURVES (1972) found that AFP levels rose in baboons during various stages of poisoning with diethylnitrosamine. Similar results were obtained by WATANABE (1971), who induced hepatomas in rats with 4-dimethylazobenzene. Alpha globulin appeared in the serum of 76% of the rats three weeks after the animals were first given the drug; 91% of these rats developed hepatomas after 19 weeks.

Determination of AFP levels can help differentiate chorioepithelioma and hydratidiform mole from normal pregnancy (SEPPÄLÄ et al., 1972). Hormonal tests are positive in all such cases; AFP is elevated only when a fetus is present.

ELGORT et al. (1972) compared the sensitivity of the agaroprecipitation method for detecting AFP with immunoradioautography, a more sensitive method. Sera collected from patients in five African countries (Uganda, Nigeria, Senegal, Kenya, and the Congo), from Jamaica, Singapore, and the USSR were investigated by both methods. The increased sensitivity of the second technique resulted in the transfer of a considerable proportion of the hepatomas from the AFP-negative to the AFP-positive group. By agaroprecipitation, 75% of the African hepatocellular carcinoma patients were found positive and 64% of the Soviet patients. The more sensitive technique detected AFP in more than half of the previously negative sera, so that a positive reaction was detected in sera from 89.2% of the African and 87.1% of the Soviet patients. However, the specificity of the reaction decreased: 20% of the African controls were positive and 6% of the USSR controls. False positive reactions in Soviet patients were almost exclusively connected with liver diseases, as were those in patients from Uganda, Kenya, and Singapore, but not for those from the Congo and Senegal.

Table 7. Comparison of positive AFP test in hepatoma and non-hepatoma patients in various laboratories (STILLMANN and ZAMCHECK, 1970)

Author	Number of cases	Hepatoma		Non-hepatoma	
		Number	% pos.	Number	% pos.
ABELEV, 1967	308	28	60.7	280	3.5
SMITH and TODD, 1968	402	32	59.3	370	0
PURVES, 1968	194	133	75.2	YY	1.6
URIEL et al., 1968	3902	112	79.4	3790	0.02
ALPERT et al., 1968	262	40	50	193	1
TOLI et al., 1969	262	35	40	227	0
Total	5330	380	68.1	4907	0.3

The results of various investigators' attempts to detect AFP are summarized in Tables 7 and 8. The radioimmunoassay is so sensitive that levels of AFP as low as 2 ng/ml of serum can be detected. Such low levels are present in most healthy persons. The diagnostic value of this technique lies not in its ability to detect AFP, but in the level of AFP it can detect. The serological test for AFP is valuable in the diagnosis of hepatomas. Its accuracy is surprisingly high and can be compared with that of the percutaneous liver needle biopsy and has far less risk for the patient. Disappearance of AFP helps evaluation of the patient's response to therapy. Positive levels of AFP are also found in many cases of tetratoblastomas.

CEA of the digestive tract (GOLD) have been used for diagnostic and prognostic purposes. Soon after the discovery of the antigen, GOLD reported on a patient who was clinically healthy but whose serum exhibited a positive reaction for CEA. When a laparatomy was performed, a very small primary tumor was found; histological examination showed it to be an adenocarcinoma. NORLAND et al. (1969) observed that colon carcinomas could be distinguished from normal colon and inflammatory conditions of the colon with immunofluorescent staining and precipitin inhibition tests. The greatest amount of information concerning the diagnostic and prognostic value of digestive tract CEA has come from the extensive studies of ZAMCHECK et al. (MOORE et al., 1971a, b; ZAMCHECK, 1972a, b; STILLMAN and ZAMCHECK, 1970). In the first three months of 1971, they tested about 1,000 sera using the radioimmunoassay method of THOMPSON et al. (1969) und reagent supplied by GOLD. They confirmed that a small amount of CEA could be detected in sera of patients

Table 8. Diagnostic value of AFP for detection of liver carcinoma

Author	Diagnosis	Method	Number of cases	% pos.
Abelev (1967)	Primary liver cancer	DD	28	60
	Hepatocellular cancer	DD	18	77
	Metastatic liver tumor	DD	67	0
	Testicular tumor	DD	47	21
	Liver diseases	DD	60	0
Masopust et al., (1968)	Teratoma	DD	7	57
	Hepatocellular cancer	DD	3	33
	Other tumors	DD	138	0
Smith (1971)	Primary hepatoma	DD	10	50
	Primary hepatoma	CEP	10	90
	Embryonal testicular cancer	DD	20	25
	Embryonal testicular cancer	CEP	20	70
	Hepatitis	DD	15	0
	Hepatitis	CEP	15	0
	Pregnant women[a]			
	1st trimester	CEP	10	0
	2nd trimester	CEP	11	27
	3rd trimester	CEP	10	80
Smith and O'Neill (19yy)	Embryonal cell cancer testis	DD	15	27
	Embryonal carcinoma testis	DD	5	40
	Seminoma	DD	5	0
	Choriocarcinoma of the ovary	DD	6	0
	Dermoid cyst	DD	5	0
	Primary hepatoma Hong Kong	DD	60	65
	Primary hepatoma USA	DD	19	42
	Infectious hepatitis		170	0
	Cirrhosis		110	0
	Leukemia		120	0
	Pregnancy		104	0
	Normal		100	0

[a] All negative in DD. DD = double diffusion, CEP = counter electrophoresis.

with colonic and pancreatic tumors. CEA was also detected in patients with types of cancer other than those of the digestive tract and in some patients without cancer. Summarizing their results in histologically proven cases, they found: 72% of 60 patients with colonic cancer exhibited a positive reaction; 88% of 26 patients with advanced pancreatic cancer were positive; 39% of 28 patients with other diseases of the digestive tract were positive. Positive reactions were found in most patients with lung and breast cancer. There was an interesting correlation between the amount of detectable CEA with diagnosis and stage of the disease. Two positive patients with benign polyps also had liver cirrhosis; they remained positive after surgical removal of the polyps. The results are summarized in Table 9.

The fate of CEA after operation was followed in 19 patients. Six patients with no known metastases were positive preoperatively and were all negative at least 7 days postoperatively. Five patients, negative preoperatively, remaind negative after the operation. Five preoperatively positive patients remained positive after palliative operation, but the level of CEA changed. In two cases, in which the disease was progressing despite the operation, the negative reaction changed to a positive one. From a prognostic point of view, interesting results were obtained from 7 patients on whom the assay was done 2 weeks to 2 years after surgery. The results are shown in Table 10.

Table 9. Finding of CEA in various groups of cancer patients
(MOORE *et al.*, 1971)

	No. of patients	% positive
Normal control	44	0
Patients with cancer		
Colonic	60	72
Pancreatic	26	88
Other Gl	28	39
Non Gl	25	36

Table 10. Fate of CEA in patients with cancer of colon in relation to operation
(MOORE *et al.*, 1971)

	Pre-operative	Post-operative
5	+	+
6[a]	+	—
5	—	—
2	—	+

[a] All 6 were without known metastasis.

Table 11. Finding of elevated CEA in non-tumor diseases of the digestive tract

Diagnosis	Total	Positive	% positive
Colitis	41	1	2.4
Diverticular disease	17	5	29.4
Bleeding in the GI tract	29	0	0
Liver disease	111	47	42.3
Pancreatitis	34	12	35.3

From a diagnostic point of view, it is important to know in which other diseases this reaction is also found to be positive (Tables 11, 12). The percentage of positive findings also depends on the stage of the disease — it is highest in the most advanced cancer (Table 13) — and on whether theer is metastasis (Table 14).

BURTIN *et al.* (1972) used immunofluorescence and specific anti-CEA serum to detect CEA in the colonic mucosa of 48 young children. In all cases, including two children over 7 years old, the reaction was positive.

Using radioimmunoassay, MARTIN and MARTIN (1972) found CEA not only in primary adenocarcinomas of the colon and in liver metastasis but also in colonic mucosa from noncancerous diseases. CEA was not detectable in noncancerous gastric mucosa.

Table 12. CEA in various cancer and non-cancer Diseases

Diagnosis	Total	Positive	% positive
Control persons	40	0	0
Cancer of the colon	43	40	93
Cancer of the pancreas	13	13	100
Cancer of GI tract (other)	14	6	42.8
Adenocarcinoma	7	6	8
Cancer of the colon (postoperatively)	23	6	27.2
Disease of the liver	53	24	45.2
Disease of the GI	45	10	22.2
Disease of the kidney	17	7	41
Other	11	2	18
Total cancer diseases (without postoperative cases)	77	65	84.4
Total noncancerous disease	126	43	34.1

Table 13. Detectable amount of CEA of digestive tract carcinoma in relation to the diagnosis

	Total number	Number of sera showing CEA at:				
		2 ng	4 ng	6 ng	8 ng	10 ng or more
Benign polyp	15	14	0	0	1	0
Malignant polyp	5	4	1	0	0	0
Invasive carcinoma of the colon	21	9	4	2	1	5
Distant carcinoma of the colon	34	4	2	2	0	26

Table 14. Comparison of detection of CEA in colon carcinoma patients with and without metastases (MOORE et al., 1972)

	CEA pos.	CE mg	% positive
No metastases	4	44	8
With metastases	23	2	92

BURTIN et al. (1972) used an immunofluorescent technique to compare the antigenicity of 25 polyps of the colon of various histologic types. In all polyps, there was a decrease in the amount of normal cytoplasmic antigens, a decrease or even lack of the normal plasma-membrane antigens of the colonic cells, and presence of CEA of cancer of the gastrointestinal tract. From the quantitative point of view, the CEA and normal cytoplasmic antigens were more abundant in the differentiated polyps than in the undifferentiated ones. No prognostic indications can be drawn from these immunological findings. The presence of the CEA can be observed in noncancerous intestinal mucosa, including that of hemorrhoids.

Five elderly persons with diverticulitis who exhibited positive reactions were followed for a year and showed no signs of tumors. One year, however, is too short to allow any conclusions to be drawn.

It is also possible that old age is a limiting factor in interpreting the finding of CEA. ZAMCHECK quotes a personal communication from GOLD in which he says that 30 out of 70 patients clinically free of cancer but positive for CEA later developed cancer.

Positive reactions were found in 49% of patients with severe alcoholic diseases of the liver; negative reactions were found in all patients with nonalcoholic liver diseases. It was shown that CEA observed in cirrhosis is immunologically identical to CEA of cancer of the digestive tract.

Carcinomas of the stomach were usually less well differentiated than the colonic tumors. CEA was observed in the same regions as in colonic tumors, but in lower quantities than in comparable colonic cancer.

Six pancreatic cancers were studied: one well-differentiated adenocarcinoma contained a large amount of CEA, observable on the surface, in the lumina and in the cytoplasm of isolated cells. The metastases of this tumor, which were more differentiated, seemed to contain more CEA. In two moderately differentiated adeno- carcinomas, a small amount of CEA was detected on the cell surface. The other cancers were anaplastic and did not contain detectable amounts of CEA. In carcinomas of bronchus, breast, ovary and anus, no CEA was detected by this method.

GOLD (1967) found that patients with carcinoma of the digestive tract have circulating antibodies against this antigen. He found an interesting relationship between the clinical status of the tumor and the presence of antibodies: while anti- bodies were found in 70% of patients without metastatic tumors, no antibodies were found in patients with metastatic tumors. GOLD suggested that this difference may be the result of absorption of the antibodies on the mass of the tumor. This explanation is supported by the finding of such antibodies after surgical removal of the tumor in 4 patients who did not have circulating antibodies preoperatively. Observations of pregnant women ran in parallel to these results: in the second trimester antibodies against CEA were found in 9 out of 10 women, in the third trimester, in only 1 out of 10, but in 6 out of 8 women in the first week *post partum*. Healthy persons do not have these antibodies and in non-neoplastic diseases such antibodies were found in only two cases: one, a patient with partial colonectomy for diverticulitis and the second, a patient who developed a pancreatic malignancy.

Other authors did not find such antibodies in the sera of patients with cancer of the digestive tract. COLLATZ *et al.* (1971) investigated sera from 190 cancer patients, 125 of whom had cancer of the digestive tract. Using techniques similar to those of GOLD (1967), i.e. passive hemagglutination, immunoadsorption and immuno- fluorescence, they found negative results in all cases. Any detected reaction was shown to be directed against normal tissue components which were present in the extracts of the colon tumors. Similar negative results were obtained by LoGERFO *et al.* (1972) in a study which included 110 patients with non-metastatic colonic carcinomas, 122 patients with other gastrointestinal, breast and lung tumors, 20 pregnant women and 13 healthy volunteers.

Table 15. Percentage of positive CEA reaction in relation to stage of the disease (ZAMCHECK *et al.*, 1972)

Diagnosis	% positive
Early carcinoma	45
Locally invasive	55
Distant metastases	88—96

Table 16. Percentage of positive CEA reaction as detected in various laboratories (ZAMCHECK *et al.*, 1972)

Laboratory	Total of cases	% positive
Montreal	36	97
Boston (1)	35	91
Boston (2)	60	72
New York	101	86
Buffalo	33	82

Table 17. CEA assay in patients whose investigations have not disclosed cancer (MOORE *et al.*, 1971)

Patient group	No. of Patients	Results	
		positive	negative
Liver disease	53		
Alcoholic	46	24	22
non-alcoholic	7	7	0
Gastrointestinal disease	45		
Colititis	8	1	7
Polyps	9	1	8
Other	28	8	20
Renal disease	17		
Ondialysis	12	6	6
Post-kidney transplant	5	1	4
Other	11	2	9

In another study, ZAMCHECK's group examined sera from 279 persons (Table 15). In the case of liver diseases, only those patients with alcoholic liver disease gave positive results (24 out of 46 = 52%). ZAMCHECK compared the percentage of positive results obtained in various laboratories and compiled the information given in Table 16. His comparison of colonic cancer at various stages (Table 17) should be noted.

An antigen which cross-reacts with CEA was found in mucinous ovarian fluid (MᶜNEIL *et al.*, 1969).

LoGERFO *et al.* (1971) examined sera and plasma from 674 patients using the radioimmunoassay. Elevated levels of CEA were observed in 87 patients out of 101 with colon carcinoma, in 30 out of 45 patients with breast cancer, in 26 out of 35 patients with lung carcinoma and in 20 out of 51 patients with prostatic carcinoma. Positive levels were also found in 11 out of 299 patients with various diseases other than neoplastic ones. Two of these since developed malignancies, one a hepatoma and the other, lung carcinoma.

As mentioned previously, follow-up of CEA levels seems to be very important in evaluating the postoperative period. GOLD (THOMPSON, 1969), MOORE (1971), DGAR (1971), LoGERFO (1971) and REYNOSO (1972) found that the positive reaction quickly fell postoperatively to negative levels. Reappearance of a positive reaction is always a warning of the possible recurrence of the malignant disease.

In conclusion, I shall quote ZAMCHECK *et al.*, since they have the most experience in diagnostic and prognostic evaluation of CEA:

„The methods used for preparation and detection of CEA are highly complex and do not yet lend themselves to the routine usage possible with the alpha-fetoglobulin test. It appears that malignant may be differentiated from nonmalignant processes in part by the amount of CEA-like substance found in the serum. The present low serum threshold positivity (2.5 ng/ml is generally used) misses fewer cancers at the price of reporting more false positive assays. By setting a higher threshold (for example greater than 5 ng/ml), greater reliability of the positive diagnosis is achieved at the price of missing some cancers. The serum assay for CEA detects cancer of the colon with a high degree of reliability. This assay may prove useful in predicting persistence or recurrence of tumor after resection of colonic carcinoma. The same assay detects adenocarcinoma of the pancreas with promising regularity. The assay must be cautiously interpreted in patients with alcoholic liver diseases and with renal failure. Further studies are needed to determine whether the CEA assay detects digestive tract malignancy early enough to improve prognosis."

Gastric sulphoglycoproteins have been less extensively studied than AFP or CEA of the digestive tract. HAAKINEN and VIKARI (1969) found that this antigen was present in the gastric juice of 96% of patients with gastric cancer. In 24 patients who survived 5 years postoperatively, this antigen was found in only 17%. In patients with various gastric diseases, a positive reaction was found in 9.4%; 14% of patients with peptic ulcer were also positive. The latter finding limits the usefulness of this test for diagnosis. On the other hand, a negative test for FSA (as the authors suggested it be called) in a patient with an ulcer may help exclude cancer of the stomach.

Ascertaining the fate of normal surface antigens offers an interesting approach to cancer diagnosis. Two studies concerning cancer of the digestive tract will be mentioned in this connection. SHEAHAN *et al.* (1971) found that A, B and H antigens, which can normally be detected in the mucosa of the stomach and small intestine, were diminished or absent in eight out of nine patients with gastric epithelial malignancies. In all metastases, these antigens were not found at all. BURTIN *et al.* (1971) studied 10 colonic adenocarcinomas and 10 colonic polyps, samples of normal colonic mucosa, 3 fetal intestines and colonic tumors maintained in organ culture (WOLFF and WOLFF, 1966). A membrane-associated antigen(s) of the normal colonic mucosa was not detected in the carcinomas and the level was decreased in the colonic polyps. There seems to be a correlation between the reappearance of CEA and loss of the normal membrane antigen.

2. Prospective Immunotherapeutic Uses of Carcinoembryonic Antigens

Theoretically, there are at least two ways to utilize a cancer-specific antigen in immunotherapy: 1) directly, for passive and active immunization or 2) indirectly, in the preparation of specific antibodies to which an anticancer drug could be bound. In the latter case, the antibodies would assure a higher concentration of the drug in the cancer tissue, thus leaving the level in normal tissue at a harmless level. The second approach sounds very promising, and could utilize any of the highly purified antigens. No other cancer-specific antigen, including those from the tumor systems in animals, has been purified to the extent as AFP and CEA of the digestive tract; highly specific antibodies which do not cross-react with normal tissue are available against these antigens.

The applicability of the first approach — active or passive immunization — does not appear to be so remote. Thus far, however, only one of the described antigens — transplantation CEA — could possibly be used. Immunity to the other CEA's does not appear to influence tumor growth. Even GOLD's CEA, which is an extra-cellular product closely related to the cell membrane, does not show promising indications that it could be used to stimulate active or passive immunity against cancer. GOLD himself could not find any relation between humoral anti-CEA antibodies and the clinical status and course of cancer of the digestive tract (GOLD, 1967). Host resistance against a tumor is more a function of cell-mediated immunity than of humoral antibodies. For this reason, GOLD (LEJTENYI *et al.*, 1971) studied the response of lymphocytes from patients with gastrointestinal cancer by observing lymphocyte transformation upon *in-vitro* exposure to the antigen. No significant response was obtained with lymphocytes from patients with gastrointestinal cancer, pregnant women or normal individuals. Thus no evidence for cell-mediated immunity against CEA was detected.

When AFP was first detected in mouse hepatomas, ABELEV *et al.* used the first purified material for active immunization. No effect of this immunization was detected in syngeneic mice subsequently grafted with the hepatoma cells. Similarly, there is no evidence from clinical observations that AFP plays any role from an immunological point of view in the growth of AFP-producing tumors. One should also keep in mind that not all cells of hepatocellular carcinoma produce AFP.

As far as I know, no one has yet used CEA of the transplantation type from intestinal tumor in immunotherapeutic trials for selected patients, despite some encouraging clinical data. This is understandable because during immunization against a tumor, there is always the possibility of provoking enhancement. Although the enhancement phenomenon has been known from the beginning of this century, its mechanism is not yet fully understood. It is not known under what conditions enhancement will not occur nor is a method of preventing formation of enhancing antibodies known. The experiments of HEPPNER and CALABRESI (1971) offer some hope — they showed that for experimental tumors, a certain dose of cytosine arabinoside selectively suppresses formation of enhancing (blocking) antibodies without suppressing cell-mediated immunity.

In experimentally induced tumors, the most clearly demonstrated case of immunity against CEA was shown for SV$_{40}$-induced tumors (see p. 23). The transplantation type of CEA was also described in polyoma-induced tumors (PEARSON and FREEDMAN, 1968). On the other hand, TING (1968) obtained negative results with polyoma-induced tumors. BLAIR (1970) also could not demonstrate CEA of the transplantation type in the so-called spontaneous mammary tumors. Some cross-reactivity between embryonic tissue and methylcholanthrene-induced tumors was observed by PREHN (1967). Intermediate between experimental tumor studies and clinical observations stand the experiments of BUTTLE (p. 22), who grew human tumors (adapted by TOOLAN) in cortisone-treated and irradiated rats. He showed that the growth of such tumors can be more effectively inhibited by immunization with human embryonic tissue than with human adult tissue.

In clinical tumors, there are observations from the HELLSTRÖMS (1970) and from our laboratory (KOLDOVSKY et al., 1972) that lymphocytes from patients with adenocarcinoma of the colon inhibit *in-vitro* growth of cells derived from these tumors. Cells derived from embryonic intestine are similarly inhibited. That natural immunity can play a role in the fate of patients with tumors of the digestive tract is supported indirectly, mainly by histological studies. YOON (1959) showed that lymphocytes and eosinophil infiltration is a favorable prognostic sign in patients with cancer of the stomach. BLACK et al. (1954, 1956, 1971) made similar observations. Lymphoreticuloendothelial reactivity was most often expressed in the form of lymphoid infiltration in the primary tumor and of follicular hyperplasia of the regional lymph nodes. This reaction is prognostically significant: 68% of patients exhibiting the reaction survived for a 5-year period; only 25% of those in whom no reaction was detectable survived the 5-year period.

Another piece of indirect evidence came from statistical data. The incidence of various tumors in two groups of women was compared: nuns and married (multiparous?) women (p. 23). The total mortality rate from cancer was somewhat lower for the nuns than for the married women. On the other hand, cancer of the larger intestine appeared among nuns with excess frequency. Mortality from this cancer was 38.6% in nuns, as compared with 22.6% in white American females. Although there may be many nonimmunological reasons for this difference, an immunologist, in connection with the finding that pregnant women react against their own embryos (HELLSTRÖM et al., 1969; GOLD, 1967), can speculate that pregnancy produces a certain degree of protection against a tumor, which shares with embryonic tissue some antigens of the transplantation type.

Thus far CEA of the transplantation type for human tumors has been described only in cancer of the digestive tract. However, there is no reason to believe that this type of CEA is limited only to this type of tumor. What is needed is a large comparative study with as many human tumors as possible of the antigenicity of different embryonic tissues (organs) at various stages of embryonic development. It would not be surprising to find that almost every tumor has its antigenic counterpart in an embryonic organ. Once the danger of enhancement is eliminated, the immunotherapy of tumors by active immunization with corresponding embryonic tissue could start almost immediately.

VIII. Appendix: Methods of Detection, Separation and Purification of Carcinoembryonic Antigens

Although the purification and characterization of normal or tumor-specific transplantation antigens are currently the center of interest in many laboratories, the problems involved have not yet been satisfactorily worked out. Purification and characterization of transplantation CEA have not yet begun.

CEA is detected by basically the same methods used for detection of any cell membrane-associated antigen. The only reliable test for detection of CEA in experimental tumors is the transplantation test in which animals are preimmunized with various materials (tumors of embryonic origin) and then challenged with living tumor cells. Changes in the pattern of tumor growth are indicative of whether some degree of immunity was obtained. The *in-vitro* cytotoxic reaction, which also can be used with human tumors, mediated either by immune cells or by serum, probably detects transplantation antigens. Thus when antiserum is prepared against embryonic tissue and properly absorbed so that it specifically reacts only with given embryonic tissue and is then also cytotoxic for tumor cells, one might assume that these embryonic tissue and cancer share a CEA of the transplantation type.

Membrane fluorescence and binding of antibodies detected by ^{125}I-labeled anti-gammaglobulin antibodies are less certain methods for detecting transplantation antigens. With these methods, any surface antigen, even one which does not elicit the transplantation reaction, can cause a positive reaction.

Animals immunized with morphological and biochemical fractions prepared from the cells containing embryonic antigens are subsequently tested with tumor (or normal) tissue containing the antigen in question. The fraction containing the antigen specifically preimmunizes the animals against the subsequent graft. This procedure has been used repeatedly for characterization of normal and tumor-specific transplantation antigens, and the best that can be said is that these antigens are found in the microsomal fraction and that they contain lipoproteins. The safest definition of a transplantation antigen is that it is a lipoprotein with mucopolysaccharide components.

The other CEA's, on the other hand, have been purified to a high degree because they represent relatively simple compounds.

1. Alpha Fetoprotein

In the early 60's, ABELEV attempted to purify by immunodiffusion this antigen which he detected in mouse hepatoma. The antigenic composition of a hepatoma is quite complex. He adapted a method of immunofiltration used for bacterial antigens to purify tissue antigens (ABELEV and ZILBER, 1968). The discovery that this antigen was antigenically identical with fetal protein made its isolation in a pure form relatively simple. The antigen — alpha globulin — is prepared from the fetal serum rather than from the tumor. For example RUOSLAHTI and SEPPÄLÄ (1971) purified the antigen according to the following procedure: The fetal serum (1.5 ml) was fractionated by electrofocusing in a pH gradient from pH 4 — 6. A precipitin was formed when the serum sample was mixed with the less dense Ampholine solution. The fetoprotein fractions were pooled and separated once more by electrofocusing. A sheep was immunized with the purified AFP and the antiserum obtained was absorbed with lyophilized normal adult human serum at a ratio of 0.2 mg: 1 ml. The monospecific antiserum was then used for immunochemical purification of the alpha-fetoprotein from larger quantities of fetal serum or from water-soluble extracts of whole fetuses. The immunoprecipitate produced by mixing the sheep antiserum with the fetal material, was washed, and the antigen-antibody complexes were separated from each other by gel filtration on Sephadex G-200 columns at pH 2.5 in 0.3 M sodium citrate buffer.

The several methods currently used to detect AFP differ markedly in sensitivity. Agaroprecipitation (Ouchterlony technique), which is the most simple and least sensitive method, can detect about 1 mg/ml. AFP can be detected directly in the section of the tumor by immunofluorescence (ENGELGARDT et al., 1971). Sandwich counter-electrophoresis (SMITH and TODD, 1968) is a more sensitive method for detecting AFP in serum. An initial counter-electrophoresis is done with rabbit antiserum in the anodic wells and test serum in the well near the cathode. After one hour all remaining fluid is removed from the wells and sheep antirabbit IgG is placed in the anodic wells. Electrophoresis is run for an additional 45 min. Precipitin bands were visible after 2 — 3 hours of incubation at room temperature. AFP at a concentration of 100 ng/ml could be detected with this procedure.

An even more sensitive method is the radioimmunoassay, with which levels as low as 2.5 ng/ml can be detected, i.e. this technique is 40,000 times more sensitive than the initial immunodiffusion technique. RUOSLAHTI and SEPPÄLÄ (1971 b) used the following procedure: Purified AFP was iodinated by the modified method of GREENWOOD et al. (1963). Sephadex G 25 was used to separate the labeled protein from the excess of free iodine. The fractions were collected in a bovine serum albumin solution (0.05% BSA). Aliquots of each fraction were counted on a gamma counter. The fraction containing 97% or more of the labeled AFP was used in the assay. Bovine serum albumin was added to a final concentration of 0.125% and the product was stored at 4 °C. After two weeks the preparation was refractionated on the Sephadex G-25 column. This labeled AFP was precipitated by specific anti-AFP antibodies at various dilutions and the antibody concentration binding 25% of the precipitated counts was selected for the inhibition tests. The standard inhibition curve was obtained by twofold dilution of standard AFP in 0.125% bovine serum albumin. Then 100 ml of 1:1 anti-AFP antiserum (1:10,000) and normal sheep serum was added and finally the labeled AFP. The test was continued as described above. The counts detected in the preparation of this tube were subtracted as non-specific radioactivity from the counts in the radioimmunoassay experiment. The serum samples were analyzed by replacing the standard dilution with an equal amount of the serum dilution.

2. CEA of the Digestive Tract (GOLD)

The first material in which GOLD and FREEDMAN (1965) detected CEA was an extract obtained from mechanically disrupted and sonicated tumor. KRUPEY *et al.* (1968), when studying the physicochemical properties of this CEA, prepared it in purified form. The tumor was first homogenized — 1000 g tissue in 2 l of distilled water in a VirTis chemimixer at 15,000 rpm. To this was added an equal volume of 1.2 M perchloric acid, and the suspension was centrifuged at 2,000 rpm. The sediment was discarded, and the supernatant was dialyzed against tap water for 24 hours and evaporated to a volume of 200 ml. The suspension was centrifuged at 35,000 rpm for 30 min, and the clear supernatant was dialyzed against distilled water, filtered through 0.22 millipore filters and lyophilized. Initial separation of the components of the lyophilized material was performed by paper-block electrophoresis. The zones containing CEA activity were suspended in 5 ml of distilled water. This material was then dialyzed against distilled water and lyophilized. Identical zones from the paper-block electrophoretogram were prepared in the same way from the extract of normal tissue. The fractions obtained by the electrophoretic procedure were chromatographed on Sephadex G-200. Those fractions possessing CEA activity, as well as corresponding fractions of normal tissue samples, were dialyzed against distilled water.

To detect CEA, GOLD and FREEDMAN originally used antisera produced in rabbits tolerant to normal tissue extract and immunized with tumor extracts. The specificity of these antisera was further assured by absorption with normal tissue extracts. Such specific antisera were then reacted in agaroprecipitation against samples of tissue extracts or sera.

The second technique was hemagglutination of rabbit erythrocytes with antigen covalently coupled to them with bis-diazotized benzidine (SCHON, 1959). Passive cutaneous anaphylaxis was performed in the mice according to HALPERN *et al.* (1963). Intracutaneous injection of 0.02 ml of the test serum was followed three hours later by intravenous injection of 1 mg of test antigen in 0.3 ml of 0.2% trypan blue. The reaction was read 30 minutes later by sacrificing the animals and measuring the diameter of the largest subcutaneous dye spot.

All of these techniques have relatively low sensitivity, so the same authors later developed the radioimmunoassay (THOMPSON *et al.*, 1969). The purified antigen was labeled with radioactive iodine by the method of HUNTER and GREENWOOD (1964). The ^{125}I-CEA was separated from the unreacted ^{125}I by dialyzing against distilled water. The radioimmunoassay is based on a modification of the coprecipitation-inhibition technique of FARR (1958), whereby one first obtains a standard inhibition curve using standard CEA. This curve is then compared with inhibition curves produced by the samples under investigation. Another method, which also uses a coprecipitation-inhibition assay, was suggested by HANSEN *et al.* (1971). Zirconyl phosphate gel is used for precipitation. Both methods yielded equal results in analysis of patient serum or plasma (KUPCHIK *et al.*, 1972).

EGAN *et al.* (1972) suggested the use of the triple-isotope double-antibody technique to detect CEA. Three gamma emitters were used: ^{125}I to follow the precipitation of CEA, ^{131}I for precipitation of goat anti-CEA by horse antigoat IgG and ^{22}Na as a volume marker (which eliminates the need to wash the precipitate).

The CEA was labeled by the chloramine-T method mentioned previously (see p. 52). The goat anti-IgG was labeled with [131]I. In the double-antibody technique, it is important to have complete precipitation of the primary antibodies by the secondary (precipitating) antibodies. The goat antiserum must be tested to determine the optical precipitating conditions. The assay for CEA is based on the inhibition by CEA of the bonding of approximately 0.5 ng of CEA labeled with ^{125}I by an amount of goat anti-CEA to bind 30—40% of this amount. The standard curve for inhibition of precipitation of ^{125}I-CEA is obtained by adding standard CEA in twofold dilution to 10 µl of 0.5 ng ^{125}I-CEA, an amount of [22]Na to give 50,000 cpm, goat anti-IgG-^{131}I to give 20,000 cpm, 200 µl PBSR, 50 µl of goat anti-CEA diluted in normal goat serum to bind 30 — 40% of the CEA. After 2 hours, 100 µl of horse antigoat IgG is added, after an additional 45 minutes incubation at 37 °C, and 15 min at 4 °C, the samples are centrifuged, all but about 20 µl of the supernatant is removed and the sediment counted. The entire assay can be done without changing the container.

IX. References

Abelev, G. I.: Study of the antigenic nature of tumors. Acta Un. int. Cancer 19, 80 (1963).

Abelev, G. I.: Production of embryonal alfa-globulin by hepatomas. Review of experimental and clinical data. Cancer Res. 28, 1344 (1968).

Abelev, G. I., Asceritova, I. V., Kitajevskij, N. A., Perova, S. D., Perevodchikova, N. I.: Embryonal serum alfa-globulin in cancer patients — diagnostic value. Int. J. Cancer 2, 551 (1967).

Abelev, G. I., Avenirova, Z. A.: (In Russian). Prob. Onkol. 6, 57 (1960).

Abelev, G. I., Perova, S. D., Kramkova, N. I., Postnikova, Z. A., Irlin, I. S.: Production of embryonal alfa-globulin by transplantable mouse hepatomas. Transplant. Bull. 1, 174 (1963).

Abelev, G. I., Tsvetkov, V. S., Biryulina, T. I.: Assessment of the use of highly sensitive methods of determining alpha-feto-protein for the diagnosis of hepatocellular cancer and teratoblastoma. Biull. eksp. Biol. Med. 4, 75 (1971). (In Russian.)

Alexander, P., Hall, J. G.: The role of immunoblasts in host resistance and immunotherapy of primary sarcoma. Advanc. Cancer Res. 13, 1 (1970).

Alexander, P.: Foetal "antigens" in cancer. Nature (Lond.) 235, 137 (1972).

Albert, F., Lejeune, G., Moureau, P., Adidu, A.: Biological problem of grafting, p. 369. Eds.: Albert, F., Medawar, P. B. Université de Liège 1959.

Alpert, E., Michl, J., de Nechaud, B.: Alpha-1-fetoglobulin in the diagnosis of human hepatoma. New Engl. J. Med. 278, 984 (1968).

Alpert, E., Zuckerman, J.: Absence of alpha-fetoprotein antigen or antibody in maternal sera. Lancet 1970 II, 465.

Alpert, E., Schur, P., Drysdale, J., Isselbacher, K.: Human alpha-1-fetoprotein: purification and physical properties. Fed. Proc. 30, 246 (1971).

Amos, D. B., Cohen, I., Klein, W. J.: Mechanism of immunologic enhancement. Transplant. Proc. 2, 68 (1971).

Aoki, T., Johnson, P. A.: Suppression of Gross leukemia cell surface antigens — kind of antigenic modulation. J. nat. Cancer Inst. 49, 183 (1972).

Arpels, C., Southam, C. M.: Cytotoxicity of sera from healthy persons and cancer patients. Int. J. Cancer 4, 548 (1969).

Auerbach, R.: The development of immunocompetent cells. Develop. Biol. Suppl. 1., 254 (1967).

Auerbach, R., Globerson, A.: In vitro induction of the graft versus host reaction. Exp. Cell Res. 42, 31 (1966).

Auterst, J., Sjögren, H. O.: Crossreacting TSTA in adeno 7 and 12 tumors demonstrated by ^{51}Cr cytotoxicity and isograft rejection tests. Int. J. Cancer 4, 279 (1969).

Avdeyev, G. I., Baskayev, I. S., Kogalskii, V. Y.: A study of antigens of some human tumors. In: Specific Tumor Antigens., p. 333 (Ed.: R. J. C. Harris). UICC Monograph series. Vol. 2. Copenhagen: Munksgaard 1969.

Axelrad, A. A.: Changes in the resistance to the proliferation of isotransplanted Gross virus induced lymphoma cells as measured by spleen colony assay. Nature (Lond.) 199, 80 (1963).

Baldwin, R. W.: Immunity to methylcholanthrene induced tumors in inbred rats following atrophy and regression of implanted tumors. Brit. J. Cancer 9, 682 (1955)

Baldwin, R. W., Barker, C. R.: Tumor-specific antigenicity of aminoazo-dye induced rat hepatomas. Int. J. Cancer 2, 355 (1967).

Baldwin, R. W., Glaves, D.: Delation of normal liver cell surface component from transplanted rat hepatomas. An. Rep. Brit. Europ. Cancer Camp. 46, 236 (1968).

Baldwin, R. W., Glaves, D., Vose, B. M.: Fetal antigen expression on chemically induced rat neoplasms. Embryonic and fetal antigens. Ed.: N. G. Anderson, J. Coggin, E. Cole, J. W. Holleman. Conf. 720208 USAEC. Cancer 2, 193 (1972).

BALDWIN, R. W., GLAVES, D., VOSE, B. M.: Embryonic antigenic expression in chemically induced rat hepatomas and sarcomas. Int. J. Cancer 10, 233 (1972).

BARRET, M. K., DERRINGER, M. K.: An induced adaptation in transplantable tumor of mice. J. nat. Cancer Inst. 11, 51 (1950).

BARTH, R. F., RUSSEL, P. F.: The antigenic specificity of spermatozoa. I. An immunofluorescent study of the histocompatibility antigens. J. Immunol. 93, 13 (1964).

BAUER, H., SCHÄFER, W.: Isolierung eines gruppenspezifischen Antigens aus Hühner-Myeloblastose Virus (BAI Stamm A). Z. Naturforsch. 20b, 815 (1965).

BECHWITH, J. B., MARTIN, R. F.: Observation on the histopathology of neuroblastomas. J. Pediat. Surg. 3, 106 (1968).

BECK, J. S., EDWARDS, R. G., YOUNG, M. R.: Immune fluorescence technique and the isoantigenicity of mammalian spermatozoa. J. Reprod. Fertil. 4, 103 (1962).

BEER, A. E., BILLINGHAM, R. E., YANG, S. L.: Maternally induced transplantation immunity, tolerance and runt disease in rats. J. exp. Med. 135, 808 (1972).

BEER, A. E., BILLINGHAM, R. E., HOERR, R. A.: Elicitation and expression of transplantation immunity in the uterus. Transplant. Proc. 3, 609 (1971).

BEER, A. E., BILLINGHAM, R. E., YANG, S. L.: Further evidence concerning the antigenic status of the trophoblasts. J. exp. Med. 135, 1177 (1972).

BEER, A. E., BILLINGHAM, R. E.: Maternally acquired runt disease. Science 179, 240 (1973).

BERG, J. W.: Inflammation and prognosis in breast cancer. A search for host resistance. Cancer (N.Y.) 12, 714 (1959).

BERGSTRAND, C. G., CZAR, B.: Demonstration of new protein fraction in serum from human fetus. Scand. J. clin. Lab. Invest. 8, 174 (1956).

BILL, A. H., MORGAN, A.: Evidence for immune reaction in neuroblastoma and future possibilities for investigation. J. Pediat. Surg. 5, 111 (1970).

BILLINGHAM, R. E.: Transplantation immunity and maternal-fetal relation. New Engl. J. Med. 270, 667 (1970).

BILLINGHAM, R. E., BRENT, L., MEDAWAR, P. B.: Actively acquired tolerance of foreign cells. Nature 172, 603 (1953).

BILLINGHAM, R. E., BRENT, L., MEDAWAR, P. B.: Quantitative studies on tissue transplantation immunity: III. Actively acquired tolerance. Phil. Trans. (B) 239, 357 (1956).

BILLINGHAM, R. E., BRENT, L.: Acquired tolerance of foreign cells in newborn animals. Proc. roy. Soc. B. 146, 78 (1956).

BILLINGHAM, R. E., LAMPKIN, G. H.: Further studies in tissue homotransplantation in cattle. J. Embryol. exp. Morph. 5, 351 (1957).

BILLINGHAM, R. E., SILVERS, W. K.: Induction of tolerance of skin isografts from male donors in female mice. Science 128, 780 (1958).

BILLINGHAM, R. E., BRENT, L., BROWN, J. B., MEDAWAR, P. B.: Time of onset and duration of transplantation immunity. Transplant. Bull. 6, 410 (1959).

BILLINGHAM, R. E., BROWN, J. B., DEFENDI, V., SILVERS, W. K., STEINMULLER, D.: Quantitative studies on the induction of tolerance of homologous tissues and runt disease in the rat. Ann. N.Y. Acad. Sci. 87, 457 (1960).

BITTNER, J. J.: A review of genetic studies on the transplantable tumors. J. Genet. 31, 471 (1935).

BJÖRKLUND, B.: In: Discussion following paper by Rapport & Graf. Cancer Res. 21, 1240 (1961).

BLACK, M. M., OPLER, S. R., SPEER, F. D.: Structural representatives of tumor host relationships in gastric carcinoma. Surg. Gynec. Obstet. 102, 599 (1956).

BLACK, M. M., OPLER, S. R., SPEER, F. D.: Microscopic structure of gastric carcinoma and their regional lymph nodes in relation to survival. Surg. Gynec. Obstet. 98, 725 (1954).

BLACK, M. M., FREEMAN, C., MORK, T., HARVEI, S., CUTLER, S. J.: Prognostic significance of microscopic structure of gastric carcinomas and their regional lymph nodes. Cancer (Philad.) 27, 703 (1971).

BLAIR, P. B.: Search for crossreacting antigenicity between mammary tumor virus induced mammary tumor and embryonic antigens: Effect of immunization on development of spontaneous mammary tumors. Cancer Res. 30, 1199 (1970).

BOLLAG, W.: Heterologe Transplantation von Tumoren bei Vorbehandlung der Empfangtiere mit Gewebe der Spendertiere während der Embryonalzeit. Experientia (Basel) 11, 227 (1955).

BOLLAG, W.: Immunität und Toleranz gegen heterologe Tumoren. Oncologia (Basel) 9, 233 (1956).

BORAHES, D. K., HILDEMAN, W. H.: Maturation of alloimmune responsiveness in mice. Transplantation **3**, 202 (1965).

BORSOS, T., RAPP, H. J., COLTEN, H. R.: Immune hemolysis and functional properties of second (C_2) and fourth (C_4) components of complement. I. Functional differences among C_4 sites on cell surface. J. Immunol. **105**, 1439 (1970).

BRAND, E.: Aminoacid composition of simple proteins. Ann. N.Y. Acad. Sci. **47**, 187 (1946).

BRAWN, R. J.: Possible association of embryonal antigen(s) with several primary 3-methylcholanthrene induced murine sarcomas. Int. J. Cancer **6**, 245 (1970).

BUBENIK, J., KOLDOVSKY, P.: The mechanism of antitumor immunity studied by means of transfer of immunity. Folia Biol. (Praha) **10**, 427 (1964).

BUBENIK, J., PERLMAN, P., HELMSTEIN, K., MOBERGER, G.: Immune response to urinary bladder tumors in man. Int. J. Cancer **5**, 39 (1970)

BUBENIK, J., PERLMAN, P., HELMSTEIN, K., MOBERGER, G.: Cellular and humoral responses to human urinary bladder carcinomas. Int. J. Cancer **5**, 310 (1970)

BURNET, F. M.: Principles in Animal Virology. New York: Academic Press 1960.

BURNET, F. M., FENNER, F.: The production of antibodies. McMillan Co. 1949.

BURTIN, P., BUFFE, D., v. KLEIST, S., WOLFF, E., WOLFF, M.: Mise en évidence de l'antigène carcinoembryonnaire spécifique des cancers digestifs dans les tumeurs humaines entretenues en culture organotypique. Int. J. Cancer **5**, 88 (1970).

BURTIN, P., v. KLEIST, D., SABINE, M. C.: Loss of normal colonic membrane antigens in human cancers of the colon. Cancer Res. **31**, 1038 (1971).

BURTIN, P., SABINE, M. C., CHAVANLA, G.: Presence of carcinoembryonic antigen in children's colonic mucosa. Int. J. Cancer **10**, 72 (1972).

BURTIN, P., MARTIN, E., SABINE, M. C., v. KLEIST, S.: Immunology study of polyps of the colon. J. nat. Cancer Inst. **48**, 25 (1972).

BUTTLE, G. A. H., FRYAN, A.: Effect of previous injection of homologous embryonic tissue on the growth of certain transplantable mouse tumors. Nature (Lond.) **215**, 1495 (1967).

BUTTLE, G. A. H., KELLET, O., KOVACS, N.: Memoirs of the society of Endocrinology. N. **10**, 133 (1960).

BUTTLE, G. A. H., EPERON, J. L., KOVACS, E.: An antigen of malignant and embryonic tissue. Nature (Lond.) **194**, 780 (1962).

BUTTLE, G. A. H., EPERON, J. L., MENZIES, D. N.: Induced tumor resistance in rat. Lancet **1964 II**, 12.

CATALANO, L. W., HARTER, D. H., HSU, K. C.: Common antigen in meningioma-derived cell cultures. Science **175**, 180 (1971).

CHU, E., STJERNWÄRD, J., CLIFFORD, P., KLEIN, G.: Reactivity of human lymphocytes against autochtonous and allogenic normal and tumor cells in vitro. J. nat. Cancer Inst. **39**, 595 (1967).

CHUTNA, J., HASKOVA, V.: Antigenicity of embryonic tissue. Folia Biol. (Praha) **5**, 85 (1959).

CHUTNA, J., POKORNA, Z.: IgM and IgG antibodies after immunization with organ specific testicular antigen. Folia Biol. (Praha) **13**, 68 (1967).

COGGIN, J. H., AMBROSE, K. R., ANDERSON, N. G.: Fetal antigen capable of inducing transplantation immunity against SV 40 hamster tumor cells. J. Immunol. **105**, 524 (1970).

COGGIN, J. H., AMBROSE, K. R., BELLONY, B. B., ANDERSON, N. G.: Tumor immunity in hamsters immunized with fetal tissues. J. Immunol. **107**, 526 (1971).

COHEN, A. M.: Host immunity to growing sarcomas: tumor specific serum inhibition of tumor specific cellular immunity. Cancer (Philad.) **31**, 81 (1973).

COHEN, A. M., BURDICH, J. F., KETCHAM, A. S.: Current research review: tumor specific cellular immunity. J. surg. Res. **11**, 421 (1971).

COHEN, M. W., THORBEKE, G. J., HOCHWALD, G. M., JACOBSON, E. B.: Induction of graft vs. host reaction in newborn mice by injection of newborn or adult homologous thymus cells. Proc. Soc. exp. Biol. (N.Y.) **114**, 242 (1963).

COLIGAN, J. E., LANTENSCHLEGER, J. T., EGAN, M. L., TODD, C. W.: Isolation and characterization of carcinoembryonic antigen. Immunochemistry **9**, 377 (1972).

COLLATZ, E., v. KLEIST, S., BURTIN, P.: Further investigation of circulating antibodies in colon cancer patients: On the autoantigenicity of the carcinoembryonic antigen. Int. J. Cancer **8**, 298 (1971).

O'CONNOR, G., TATARINOV, J., ABELEV, G., URIEL, J.: A collaborative study for the evaluation of a serological test for primary liver cancer. Cancer (Philad.) **25**, 1091 (1970).

CRICHTON, M., NEIL, M., LADDLE, J. N., HELMICH, W. M., TRENTELMAN, E., WENTZ, M. W.: An antiserum to ovarian mucinous cyst fluid with colon cancer specificity. Cancer Res. 29, 1535 (1969).

DALMASSO, A. P., MARTINEZ, C., SJODIN, K., GOOD, R. A.: Role of the thymus in immunobiology. Reconstitution of immunologic capacity of mice thymectomized at birth. J. exp. Med. 118, 1089 (1963).

DAVIDSOHN, I., KAVARIK, S., KEE, C. L.: A, B and O substances in gastrointestinal carcinoma. Arch. Path. 81, 381 (1966).

DEFENDI, V.: Discussion in "Crossreacting Antigens and Neoantigens", p. 117. Ed.: J. J. TRENTIN. Baltimore: The Williams & Wilkins Co. 1967.

DENK, H., TAPPEINER, G., ECKERSTORER, R., HOLZNER, J. H.: Canceroembryonic antigen (CEA) in gastrointestinal and extragastrointestinal tumors and its relationship to tumor cell differentiation. Int. J. Cancer 10, 262 (1972).

DIEHL, V., JEREB, B., STJERNSWÄRD, J., O'TOOLE, C., AHSTRÖM, L.: Cellular immunity to neuroblastoma. Int. J. Cancer 7, 277 (1971).

DIMMOCH, N. J.: New virus specific antigen in cells infected with influenza virus. Virology 39, 224 (1969).

DOLL, R., KINLEIN, M.: Immunosurveillance and cancer: epidemiological evidence. Brit. med. J. 4, 420 (1970).

DUFF, R., RAPP, F.: Reaction of serum from pregnant hamsters with surface of cells transformed by SV 40. J. Immunol. 105, 521 (1970).

DULANEY, A. D., GOLDSMITH, Y., ARNESEN, K., BRIXTON, L.: A serologic study of the cytoplasmatic fraction from the spleen of normal and leukemic mice. Cancer Res. 9, 217 (1949).

DUMONDE, D. C., WOLSTENCROFT, R. A., PANAYI, G. S., MATTHEW, M., MORLEY, J., HOWSON, W. T.: Lymphokines: nonantibody mediators of cellular immunity generated by lymphocytes activation. Nature 224, 38 (1969).

EDNAK, E. M., OLD, L. J., VRANA, M., PLAIDIS, M.: A fetal antigen associated with human neoplasia. New Engl. J. Med. 286, 1178 (1972).

EDYNAK, E. M., OLD, L. J., VRANA, M., PLAIDIS, M.: A fetal antigen associated with human neoplasia. New Engl. J. Med. 286, 1178 (1972).

EGAN, M. L., LANTENSCHLEGER, J. T., COLIGAN, J. E., TODD, C. W.: Radioimmunoassay of carcinoembryonic antigen. Immunochemistry 9, 289 (1972).

EGAN, M. L., TODD, C. W.: Carcinoembryonic antigen: Synthesis by a continuous line of adenocarcinoma cells. J. nat. Cancer Inst. 49, 887 (1972).

EGAN, M. L., COLLIGAN, J. E., LANTENSCHLEGER, J. T., TODD, C. W.: The triple isotope double antibody assays: Application to the carcinoembryonic antigen. Ed. N. G. ANDERSON, J. H. COGGIN, E. COLE, J. W. HOLLEMAN. Conf. 720208. In: "Embryonic and Fetal Antigens in Cancer" 2, 267 (1972).

EIDIDIN, M.: Transplantation antigens in the mouse. The fate of early embryo tissue transplanted to adult host. J. Embryol. exp. Morph. 12, 309 (1964).

EILBER, F. R., MORTON, D. L.: Impaired immunological reactivity and recurrence following cancer surgery. Cancer (Philad.) 25, 362 (1970).

EILBER, F. R.: Immunological studies of human sarcomas: Additional evidence suggesting an associated sarcoma virus. Cancer (Philad.) 26, 588 (1970).

ELGORT, D. A., ABELEV, G. I., O'CONNOR, G. T.: Dependence of the specificity of the serologic test for primary liver cancer in different areas of the world on the sensitivity of the method used for detecting alphafetoprotein. Int. J. Cancer 10, 331 (1972).

ENGELGARDT, N. V., GUSJEV, A. I., SHIPOVA, L. J., ABELEV, G. I.: Immunofluorescent study of alphafetoprotein in liver and liver tumors. I. Technique of localization in the tissue section. Int. J. Cancer 7, 198 (1971).

ENGELL, H. C.: Cancer cells in the blood. Ann. Surg. 149, 457 (1959).

EVANS, C. A., ITO, Y.: Antitumor immunity in the Shope papilloma-carcinoma complex of rabbits. J. nat. Cancer Inst. 36, 1161 (1966).

FARR, R. S.: A quantitative immunochemical measure of the primary interaction between BSA and antibody. J. infect. Dis. 103, 239 (1958).

FELDMAN, M., SACHS, L.: Immunogenetic properties of tumors that have acquired homotransplantability. J. nat. Cancer Inst. 20, 513 (1957).

FELDMAN, M., YAFFE, O.: Production of organ specific antibodies following an induction of tolerance to antigens to heterologous organs. Nature (Lond.) **179**, 1353 (1957).

FELLONS, M., DAUSSET, J.: Probable haploid expression of H-LA antigen in human spermatozoa. Nature (Lond.) **225**, 191 (1970).

FELTON, L. D., KAUFFMAN, G., PRESCOTT, B., OTTINGEN, B.: Studies on the mechanism of immunological paralysis induced in mice by pneumococcal polysaccharides. J. Immunol. **74**, 17 (1955).

FERNANDEZ-COLLAZO, E., THIERER, E.: Action of ABO antisera on human spermatozoa. Fertil. and Steril. **23**, 376 (1972).

FLEXNER, S., JOBLING, J. W.: Restraint in promotion of tumor growth. Proc. Soc. exp. Biol. (N.Y.) **5**, 16 (1907).

FOLI, A. K., SHERLOCH, S., ADINOLPHI, M.: Serum-alpha-1-fetoprotein in patients with liver diseases. Lancet **1969 II**, 1267.

FOSSATI, G., CANEVARI, S., PORTA, G. D., BALZARINI, G. P., VERONESI, U.: Cellular immunity to human breast carcinoma. Int. J. Cancer **10**, 391 (1972).

FOWLER, R., SCHUBERT, W. K., WEST, C. D.: Acquired partial tolerance to homologous skin grafts in the human at birth. Ann. N.Y. Acad. Sci. **87**, 403 (1960).

FRAUMENI, J., LLOYD, J. W., SMITH, E. M., WAGONER, J. K.: Cancer mortality among nuns: Role of marital status in etiology of neoplastic diseases in woman. J. nat. Cancer Inst. **42**, 455 (1969).

FREUND, J., LIPTON, M. H., THOMPSON, G. E.: Aspermatogenesis in the guinea pig induced by testicular tissue and adjuvans. J. exp. Med. **97**, 711 (1953).

FURUSAWA, M., ADACHI, H., ASAYAMA, S.: Identification of Ehrlich tumor cells agglutinogens in the cell membrane of embryonic erythroblasts in mice of mixedagglutination reaction. Exp. Cell Res. **40**, 151 (1966).

FURUSAWA, M., KOTANI, M., TAKEUCHI, H., ASAYAMA, S.: Some antigens similarities between mouse erythrocytes and Ehrlich ascites tumor cells. Nature (Lond.) **207**, 1204 (1965).

LO GERFO, P., HERTER, F. P., BENNETT, S. J.: Absence of circulating antibodies to carcinoembryonic antigens in patients with gastrointestinal malignancy. Int. J. Cancer **9**, 344 (1972).

LO GERFO, P., KRUPEY, P., HANSEN, H. J.: Demonstration of an antigen common to several varieties of neoplasia: Assay using zirconyl phosphate gel. New Engl. J. Med. **285**, 238 (1971).

GILDEN, R. V., CARP, R. I., TAGUCHI, F., DEFENDI, V.: The nature and localization of SV 40 induced complement antigen. Proc. nat. Acad. Sci. (Wash.) **53**, 684 (1965).

GINSBURG, J., DISHON, T., BLOCH, M., GROSS, J. J.: A thermostable cytotoxic factor in normal human serum active against Lanschutz ascites tumor cell. Proc. Soc. exp. Biol. (N.Y.) **107**, 235 (1961).

GITLIN, D., BIASUCCI, A.: Development of IgG, IgM, beta, c/beta a_1, C'l esterase inhibitor, ceruloplasmin, transferrin, hemopexin, alpha-2 macroglobulin and prealbumin in the human conceptus. J. clin. Invest. **48**, 1433 (1969).

GITLIN, D., BOESMAN, M.: Serum alpha-fetoprotein, albumin and gammaglobulin in human conceptus. J. clin. Invest. **45**, 1876 (1966).

GITLIN, D.: Sites of serum alpha-fetoprotein synthesis in the human and in the rat. J. clin. Invest. **46**, 1010 (1967).

GITLIN, D.: Fetus specific serum protein in several mammals and their relation to human alpha-fetoprotein. Comp. Biochem. Physiol. **21**, 327 (1967).

GOLD, P.: Circulating antibodies against carcinoembryoantigens of the human digestive system. Cancer (Philad.) **20**, 1663 (1967).

GOLD, P.: Embryonic origin of human tumor specific antigens. Progr. exp. Tumor Res. **14**, 43 (1971).

GOLD, P.: Antigenic reversion in human cancer. Ann. Rev. Med. **22**, 85 (1971).

GOLD, P., FREEDMAN, S. O.: Demonstration of tumor specific antigens in human colonic carcinomata by immunological tolerance and absorption technique. J. exp. Med. **121**, 439 (1965).

GOLD, P., FREEDMAN, S. O.: Specific canceroembryonic antigens of the human digestive system. J. exp. Med. **122**, 467 (1965).

GOLD, P., GOLD, M., FREEDMAN, S. O.: Cellular location of carcinoembryonic antigens of the human digestive system. Cancer Res. **28**, 1331 (1968).

GOLD, P., KRUPEY, J., ANSARI, H.: Position of the canceroembryonic antigen of the human digestive system on ultrastructure of tumor cell surface. J. nat. Cancer Inst. **45**, 219 (1970).

GOLDBERG, E. H., AOKI, T., BOYSE, E., BENNETT, D.: Detection of H-2 antigens on mouse spermatozoa by the cytotoxic test. Nature (Lond.) **228**, 570 (1970).

GOLDBERG, E. H., BOYSE, E. A., BENNETT, D., SCHEID, M., CARSWELL, E. A.: Serologic demonstration of H-Y (male) antigen on mouse sperms. Nature (Lond.) **232**, 478 (1971).

GOODLIN, R. C., HERZENBERG, L. A.: Pregnancy induced hemagglutinines to paternal H-2 antigens in multiparous mice. Transplant. Bull. **2**, 357 (1964).

GORER, P. A., AMOS, D. B.: Passive immunity in mice against C57 BL leukosis EL4 by means of isoimmune serum. Cancer Res. **16**, 338 (1956).

GOUDIE, R. B., MacCALLUM, H. M.: Loss of tissue specific autoantigens in thyroid tumors. Lancet **1963 II**, 1035.

GRANGER, G. A., WEISER, R. C.: Homograft target cells: Specific destruction in vitro by contact interaction with immune macrophages. Science **145**, 1425 (1964).

GREEN, H. N., GHOSE, T.: Localization of liver antibody in normal and 3'DAB treated rats. Nature (Lond.) **201**, 308 (1964).

GREENWOOD, F. C., HUNTER, W. H., GLIVER, J. S.: The preparation of ^{131}I-labelled human growth hormone of high specific radioactivity. Biochem. J. **89**, 114 (1963).

GROSS, L.: Intradermal immunization of C3H mice against sarcoma originated in animal of the same line. Cancer Res. **2**, 326 (1943).

GUSJEV, A. I., ENGLEGARDT, N. V., MASSEYOFF, R., CAMARIN, R., BASTERIS, B.: Immunofluorescence study of alpha-fetoprotein in liver and liver tumors. II. Localization of AFP in the tissue of patient with primary liver cancer. Int. J. Cancer **7**, 207 (1971).

HABEL, K.: Resistance of polyoma virus immune animals to transplanted polyoma tumors. Proc. Soc. exp. Biol. (N.Y.) **106**, 122 (1961).

HÄKKINEN, I. P. T.: An immunochemical method for detecting carcinomatous secretion from human gastric juice. Scand. J. Gastroent. **1**, 28 (1966).

HÄKKINEN, I. P. T.: Differentiation of antigenic gastric cancer sulphosaccharides from metastatic intestinal sulphopolysaccharides. Scand. J. Gastroent. **2**, 39 (1967).

HÄKKINEN, I. P. T., VIRTANEN, S.: The blood group activity of human gastric sulphoglycoproteins in patients with gastric cancer and normal controls. Clin. exp. Immunol. **2**, 669 (1967).

HÄKKINEN, I. P. T., JÄRVI, O., GRÖNROOS, J.: Sulphoglycoprotein antigens in human alimentary canal and gastric cancer. Int. J. Cancer **3**, 572 (1968a).

HÄKKINEN, I. P. T., KORKONEN, L. K., SAXEN, L.: The time of appearance and distribution of sulphoglycoprotein antigen in the human fetal alimentary canal. Int. J. Cancer **3**, 582 (1968).

HÄKKINEN, I. P. T., VIIKARI, S.: Occurrence of fetal sulphoglycoprotein antigen in the gastric juice of patients with gastric disease. Ann. Surg. **169**, 277 (1969).

HALPERN, B. N., NENCARE, T., Spector, S.: On the nature of the chemical mediator involved in the anaphylactic reaction in mice. Brit. J. Pharmacol. **20**, 389 (1963).

HAMILTON, F. G.: Immunity to malignant disease in man. Brit. med. J. **2**, 467 (1969).

HAMLIN, I. M. F.: Possible host resistance in carcinoma of the breast: a histological study. Brit. J. Cancer **22**, 383 (1968).

HAMERLYNCK, J., RÜHMKE, P.: A test for the detection of cytotoxic antibodies to spermatozoa in man. J. Reprod. Fertil. **17**, 191 (1968).

HANON, N.: Cell surface antigen induced by Venezuelan Equine Encephalomyelitis virus. Inf. and Immun. **2**, 713 (1970).

HANSEN, H. J., LANCE, K. P., KRUPEY, J.: Demonstration of an ion sensitive antigenic site on canceroembryonic antigen using zirconyl-phosphate gel. Clin. Res. **19**, 143 (1971).

HAVERBACH, B. J., DYCE, B. J.: Chemical characteristic of CEA and its presence in bronchogenic carcinoma, rhabdomyosarcoma and regional enteritis tissue. In: "Embryonic and Fetal Antigens". Ed.: N. G. ANDERSON *et al.* Cancer **2**, 241 (1972).

HASEK, M.: Vegetative Hybridization in Animals. (In Czech.). Praha: CSAV 1953.

HASEK, M.: Tolerance phenomena in birds. Proc. roy. Soc. B. **146**, 67 (1956).

HASEK, M.: Homotransplantation antigenicity of embryonic tissue. Folia biol. (Praha) **6**, 54 (1960).

HASEK, M., LENGEROVA, A., HRABA, T.: Transplantation immunity and tolerance. Advanc. Immunol. **1**, 1 (1961).

HELLSTROM, I.: A colony inhibition (CI) technique for demonstration of tumor cell destruction by lymphoid cells *in vitro*. Int. J. Cancer **2**, 65 (1967).

HELLSTRÖM, I., HELLSTRÖM, K. E., PIERCE, G. E., BILL, A. H.: Demonstration of cell bound and humoral immunity against neoblastoma cells. Proc. nat. Acad. Sci. (Wash.) **60**, 1231 (1968).

HELLSTRÖM, K. E., HELLSTRÖM, I.: Cellular immunity against tumor antigens. Advanc. Cancer Res. **12**, 167 (1969).

HELLSTRÖM, I., HELLSTRÖM, K. E., EVANS, C. A., HEPPENER, G., PIERCE, G. E., YANG, J. P. S.: Serum mediated protection of neoplastic cells from inhibition by lymphocytes immune against their tumor specific antigen. Proc. nat. Acad. Sci. **62**, 362 (1969).

HELLSTRÖM, K. E., HELLSTRÖM, I., BRAWN, J.: Abrogation of cellular immunity to antigenically foreign mouse embryonic cells by serum factors. Nature (Lond.) **224**, 914 (1969).

HELLSTRÖM, I., HELLSTRÖM, K. E., BILL, A. H., PIERCE, G. E., YANG, J. P. S.: Studies on cellular immunity to human neoblastoma cells. Int. J. Cancer **6**, 172 (1970).

HELLSTRÖM, I., HELLSTRÖM, K. E., SHEPARD, T. H.: Cell mediated immunity against antigens common to human colonic carcinomas and fetal gut epithelium. Int. J. Cancer **6**, 346 (1970).

HELLSTRÖM, I., HELLSTRÖM, K. E., SJÖGREN, H. O., WARNER, G. H.: Demonstration of cell-mediated immunity to human neoplasms of various histological types. Int. J. Cancer **7**, 1 (1971).

HELLSTRÖM, I., SJÖGREN, H. O., WARNER, G., HELLSTRÖM, K. E.: Blocking of cell mediated tumor immunity by sera from patients with growing neoplasms. Int. J. Cancer **7**, 226 (1971).

HELLSTRÖM, I., HELLSTRÖM, K. E., ALLISON, A. C.: Neonatally induced allograft tolerance may be mediated by serum born factor. Nature (Lond.) **230**, 49 (1971).

HENLE, W., HENLE, G., CHAMBERS, L.: Studies on the antigenic structure of some mammalian spermatozoa. J. exp. Med. **68**, 335 (1938).

HEPPNER, G. H., CALABRESI, P.: Suppression by cytosine arabinoside of the serum blocking factors of cell mediated immunity to syngeneic mouse mammary tumors. Symposium on Mammary Neoplasia. J. nat. Cancer Inst. **48**, 1161 (1971).

HERICOURT, J., RICHET, C.: De la sérotherapie dans le traitement du cancer. C. R. Acad. Sci. (Paris) **121**, 567 (1895).

HESLOP, R. W., KROHN, P. L., SPARROW, E. M.: Effect of pregnancy on survival of skin homografts in rabbits. J. Endocr. **10**, 325 (1954).

HIBBS, J. B., Jr., LAMBERT, L. H., Jr., REMINGTON, J. S.: Possible role of macrophage mediated nonspecific cytotoxicity in tumor resistance. Nature (Lond.) New Biol. **235**, 48 (1972).

HIBBS, J. B., Jr., LAMBERT, L. H., REMINGTON, J. S.: In vitro nonimmunologic destruction of cell with abnormal growth characteristic by adjuvant activated macrophages. Proc. Soc. exp. Biol. (N.Y.) **139**, 1049 (1972).

HIBBS, J. R., Lambert, L. H., REMINGTON, J. S.: Control of cancerogenesis: A possible role of the activated macrophage. Science **177**, 988 (1972).

HIRAMOTO, R., Nungester, W. J.: Penetration of serum globulins into mouse tumors. Cancer Res. **18**, 27 (1958).

HIRAMOTO, R., BERNECKY, J., JURANDOWSKY, J., PRESSMAN, D.: Immunohistochemical staining properties of the 2N-FAA rat hepatoma. Cancer Res. **21**, 1372 (1961).

HIRAMOTO, R., JURANDOWSKY, J., BERNECKY, J., PRESSMAN, D.: Lack of staining testicular tumors by anti-sperma and anti-testis antibodies. Proc. Soc. exp. Biol. (N.Y.) **111**, 505 (1962).

HIRST, A. F., BERGMAN, R. T.: Carcinoma of the prostate in men 80 or more years old. Cancer (Philad.) **7**, 136 (1954).

HIRSFELD, L., HALBER, W.: Untersuchungen über Verwandtschaftsreaktionen zwischen Embryonal- und Krebsgewebe. I. Rattenembryonen und Menschentumoren. Z. Immun.-Forsch. **75**, 193 (1932).

HIRSFELD, L.: Menschenkrebs. Z. Immun.-Forsch. **75**, 209 (1932).

HOLLINGSHEAD, A., GLEW, D., BURMAG, B., GOLD, P., HERBERMAN, R.: Skin reactive soluble antigen from intestinal cancer cell membranes and relationship to carcinoembryonic antigen. Lancet **1970 I**, 191.

HOLLINGSHEAD, A., McWRIGHT, C. G., ALFORD, T. C., GLEW, D. H., GOLD, P., HERBERMAN, R.: Separation of skin reactive intestinal cancer antigen from the carcinoembryonic antigen of Gold. Science **177**, 887 (1972).

HOLMES, E. C., MORTON, D. L., SCHIDLOVSKY, G., TRAHAN, E.: Cross reacting tumor specific transplantation antigens in methylcholanthrene induced guinea pig sarcomas. J. nat. Cancer Inst. **46**, 693 (1971).

HOUGHTON, G.: Extraction of H-2 antigen from mouse tumor cells. Transplantation **2**, 251 (1964).

HOUGHTON, G.: Moloney virus induced tumors of mice: Measurement in vitro of specific antigen. Science **147**, 506 (1965).

HRABA, T.: Mechanism and Role of Immunological Tolerance. Basel-New York: S. Karger 1968.

HRABA, T., HASEK, M., CUMLIVSKI, B.: Immunological approximation of sheep triplets, natural embryonic parabionst. Folia Biol. (Praha) **2**, 276 (1956).

HUEBNER, R. J., *et al.*: Group specific (GS) antigen expression of the C-type RNA virus genom during embryogenesis: Implication for ontogenesis and oncogenesis. Proc. nat. Acad. Sci. (Wash.) **67**, 366 (1970).

HUEBNER, R. J., ROWE, W. P., LANE, W. T.: Oncogenic effect in hamsters of human adenovirus type 12 and 18. Proc. nat. Acad. Sci. (Wash.) **48**, 2051 (1962).

HUEBNER, R. J., ROWE, W. P., TURNER, H. C., LANE, W. T.: Specific adenovirus CF antigen in virus free hamster and rat tumors. Proc. nat. Acad. Sci. (Wash.) **50**, 379 (1963).

HUEBNER, R. J., ARMSTRONG, D., OKUYAN, M., SARMA, P. S., TURNER, H. C.: Specific complement fixing viral antigens in hamster and guinea pig tumors induced by the Schmidt-Ruppin strain of avian sarcoma virus. Proc. nat. Acad. Sci. (Wash.) **51**, 742 (1964).

HULL, E. W., CARBONE, P. C., GITLIN, D., O'GARA, R. W., KELLY, M. G.: Alpha-fetoprotein in monkeys with hepatoma. J. nat. Cancer Inst. **42**, 1035 (1969).

HUMPHREY, J. H., WHITE, R. G.: Immunology for students of medicine. pp. 565—575. Philadelphia: F. A. Davis Co. 1970.

HUNTER, W. H., GREENWOOD, F. C.: A radioimmunoelectrophoretic assay for human growth hormone. Biochem. J. **91**, 43 (1964).

INBAR, M., Sachs, L.: Interaction of the carbohydrate binding protein concavalin A with normal and transformed cells. Proc. nat. Acad. Sci. (Wash.) **63**, 1418 (1969).

IVANYI, P.: The major histocompatibility antigens in various species. Current Topics in Microbiology & Immunology **53**, 1 (1970).

JOHNSON, W., JURAND, J., HIRAMOTO, R.: Immunohistologic studies on tumors containing myosin. Amer. J. Path. **47**, 1139 (1969).

KALISS, N., BRYANT, L.: Immunological enhancement. J. nat. Cancer Inst. **20**, 691 (1958).

KALISS, N., DAGG, M. K.: Immune response engendered in mice by multipartiy. Transplantation **2**, 416 (1964).

KEAST, D.: Immunosurveillance and cancer. Lancet **1970 II**, 710.

KIRBY, D. R.: Reciprocal transplantation of blastocytes between rats and mice. Nature (Lond.) **194**, 785 (1962).

KIRBY, D. R., BILLINGTON, W. S., JAMES, D. A.: Transplantation of eggs to kidney and uterus of immunized mice. Transplantation **4**, 713 (1966).

KITHIER, K., MASOPUST, J., RADL, J.: Fetal alpha-globulin of bovine serum differing from fetuin. Biochem. biophys. Acta (Amst.) **160**, 135 (1968).

KLEIN, G., SJOGREN, H. O., KLEIN, E., HELLSTRÖM, K. E.: Demonstration of resistance against methylcholanthrene induced sarcomas in the primary Autochthonous host. Cancer Res. **20**, 1561 (1960).

KLEIN, G., SJOGREN, H. O., KLEIN, E.: Demonstration of host resistance against isotransplants of lymphomas induced by the Gross agent. Cancer Res. **22**, 955 (1962).

KLEIN, E., KLEIN, G.: Antibody response and leukemic development in mice inoculated neonatally with Moloney virus. Cancer Res. **25**, 851 (1965).

KLEIN, J.: Transplantation immunity to antigens of the H-1 and H-3 locus: strength, the effect of dosage, the additive effect and the development of H-3 antigens. Folia Biol. (Praha) **11**, 169 (1965).

VON KLEIST, S., BURTIN, P.: Localisation cellulaire d'un antigène embryonnaire des tumeurs coliques humaines. Int. J. Cancer **4**, 874 (1969).

VON KLEIST, S., BURTIN, P.: On the specificity of autoantibodies present in the colon of cancer patients. Immunology **10**, 507 (1966).

KLEINSMITH, L. J., PIERCE, G. B.: Multipotentiality of single embryonal carcinoma cells. Cancer Res. **24**, 1544 (1964).

KOLDOVSKY, P.: The question of the choice of method to induce antitumor immunity within a group of mice with controlled antigenic homogeneity. Folia Biol. (Praha) **7**, 115 (1961).

KOLDOVSKY, P.: Tumor Specific Transplantation Antigen. Berlin-Heidelberg-New York: Springer 1969.

KOLDOVSKY, P., AXLER, D.: Production of heterologous cytotoxic antibodies *in vitro*. Nature (Lond.) **228**, 1323 (1970).

KOLDOVSKY, P., SVOBODA, J.: On the question of the role of heterologous tolerance in possibility to immune against tumor antigen. Folia Biol. (Praha) **8**, 101 (1962).

KOLDOVSKY, P., SVOBODA, J.: On the question of the mechanism of growth of a tumor against isoimmunity. Folia Biol. (Praha) **8**, 95 (1962).

KOLDOVSKY, P., SAWICKI, W., KOPROWSKI, H.: Crossreactivity between SV 40 transformed cell surface antigen and early embryo antigen. In: "Cellular Antigens", p. 300. (Ed.: A. NOWOTNY). Berlin-Heidelberg-New York: Springer 1972.

KOLDOVSKY, P., WEINSTEIN, J., LISCHNER, H.: Appearance of embryo and organ specific antigens in human tumors. In: Applied tumor immunity, (Ed.: H. GÖTZ). Berlin: In press.

KREIDL, A., MANDL, L.: Über den Übergang der Immunohämolysine von der Frucht auf die Mutter. Wien. klin. Wschr. **18**, 611 (1904).

KRUPEY, J., GOLD, P., FREEDMAN, S. O.: Physicochemical studies of the carcinoembryonic antigens of the human digestive system. J. exp. Med. **128**, 387 (1968).

KUPCHIK, H. Z., HANSEN, H. J., SOROKIN, J. J., ZAMCHECK, N.: Comparison of radioimmunoassays for carcinoembryonic antigens. In: Embryonal and fetal antigens. Ed.: N. G. ANDERSON *et al.* In: Cancer **2**, 261 (1972).

LAMPKIN, J. M., POTTER, M.: Response to cortisone and development of cortisone resistance in cortisone sensitive lymphosarcoma of the mouse. J. nat. Cancer Inst. **20**, 1090 (1958).

LANDER, I., AHERNE, W.:. The significance of lymphocytes infiltration in neuroblastoma. Brit. J. Cancer **26**, 321 (1972).

LANDSTEINER, K.: Centr. Bakt. 1 abst. **25**, 546 (1899).

LANDSTEINER, K., LEVINE, P.: On group specific substances in human spermatozoa. J. Immunol. **12**, 415 (1926).

LANDY, M., MICHAEL, J. G., TRAPANI, R. J., ACHISTEIN, B., WOODS, W. M., SHEAR, M. J.: An antibody complement system in normal serum lethal to mouse tumor cells. Cancer Res. **20**, 1279 (1960).

LARRIES, N. L., RICHARD, L.: Pouvoir antigène du sang foetal. C. R. Soc. Biol. (Paris) **107**, 668 (1931).

LAUMAN, J. T., DINERSTEIN, J., FIKRIG, S.: Homograft immunity in pregnancy: lack of harm to fetus from sensitization of the mother. Ann. N.Y. Acad. Sci. **99**, 706 (1962).

LAY, W. H., NUSSENZWEIG, W.: Receptors for complement on leukocytes. J. exp. Med. **128**, 991 (1968).

LEHR, H.: Über gruppenspezifische Eigenschaften des menschlichen Speichels. Z. Immun.-Forsch. **66**, 175 (1930).

LEJTENYI, M. C., FREEDMAN, S. O., GOLD, P.: Response of lymphocytes from patients with gastrointestinal cancer to the carcinoembryonic antigen of the human digestive system. Cancer (Philad.) **28**, 115 (1971).

LENGEROVA, A.: Effect of irradiation during embryogenesis on the relationship between the maternal organism and the offspring from the aspect of tissue compatibility. Folia Biol. (Praha) **3**, 333 (1957).

LEVI, E., SCHECHTMAN, A. M., SHERIUS, R. S., TOBIAS, S.: Tumor specificity and immunological suppression. Nature (Lond.) **184**, 563 (1959).

LEVY, N. L., MAHALEY, M. S., DAY, E. D.: In vitro demonstration of cell mediated immunity to human brain tumors. Cancer Res. **32**, 477 (1972).

LINDER, E.: The antigenic structure of nephroblastoma. Int. J. Cancer **4**, 232 (1969).

LINDER, E., SEPPÄLÄ, J.: Localization of alpha-fetoprotein in the human fetus and placenta. Acta path. microbiol. scand. **73**, 565 (1968).

LITTLE, C. C.: Genetics of tissue transplantation in mammals. J. Cancer Res. **8**, 75 (1924).

LITTLE, C. C., Tyzzer, E. E.: Further experimental studies on the inheritance of susceptibility to transplantable tumor, carcinoma of the Japanese Waltzing Mouse. J. med. Res. **33**, 393 (1916).

LOEB, L.: On transplantation of tumor. J. med. Res. **6**, 28 (1901).

MACHBER, B. F.: Role of soluble lymphocyte mediators in malignant tumor destruction. Lancet **1971 II**, 927.

MANSON, L. A., HICKEY, C. A., PALM, J.: H-2 alloantigen content of surface membrane of mouse cells. Wistar Inst. Mono. **8**, 93 (1968).

MARR, A. G. M., OWEN, J. A., WILSON, G. S.: Studies on the growth promoting glycoprotein fraction of fetal serum. Biochim. biophys. Acta (Amst.) **63**, 276 (1962).

MARTIN, R. F., BECHWITH, M. D.: Lymphoid infiltration in neuroblastomas. Their occurrence and prognostic significance. J. Pediat. Surg. **3**, 161 (1968).

MARTIN, F., MARTIN, M. S.: Demonstration of antigens related to colonic cancer in the digestive system. Int. J. Cancer **6**, 352 (1970).

MARTIN, F., MARTIN, M. S.: Radioimmunoassay of carcinoembryonic antigen in extracts of human colon and stomach. Int. J. Cancer **9**, 641 (1972).

MARTINEZ, C., SHAPIRO, F., GOOD, R.: Induction of immunological tolerance of tissue homografts in adult mice. Ed.: M. HASEK. In: "Mechanism of Immunological Tolerance". p. 329. Praha: CSAV 1962.

MASOPUST, J., KITHIER, K., RADL, J., KOUTECKY, J., KOTAL, L.: Occurrence of fetoprotein in patients with neoplasms and nonneoplastic diseases. Int. J. Cancer **3**, 364 (1968).

MATHÉ, G., *et al.*: Active immunotherapy for acute lymphoblastic leukemia. Lancet **1969 I**, 697.

MEDAWAR, P. B., SPARROW, E. M.: Effect of adrenocortical hormones, adrenocorticotropic hormone and pregnancy on skin transplantation in mice. J. Endocr. **14**, 240 (1956).

METCHNIKOFF, E.: Recherches sur l'influence de l'organisme sur les toxines. Sur la spermatoxine et antispermatoxine. Ann. Inst. Pasteur **14**, 1, 547 (1900).

MITCHISON, N. A.: Passage of antibodies into the intestine in the intestine in rabbits. Quart. J. exp. Physiol. **38**, 139 (1953).

MITCHISON, N. A.: Effect on offspring of maternal immunization in mice. J. Genet. **51**, 406 (1953).

MOLLER, E.: Isoantigenic properties of tumors transgressing histocompatibility barriers of the H-2 system. J. nat. Cancer Inst. **33**, 979 (1964).

MOLLER, E.: Antagonistic effect of humoral antibodies on the in vitro cytotoxicity of immune lymphoid cells. J. exp. Med. **122**, 11 (1965).

MÖLLER, G.: Studies on the development of the H-2 isoantigenic system in embryonic and newborn mice. J. Immunol. **86**, 56 (1960).

MÖLLER, G.: Phenotypic expression of isoantigen of the H-2 system in embryonic and newborn mice. J. Immunol. **90**, 271 (1963).

MÖLLER, G.: Effect of tumor growth in syngeneic recipients of antibodies against tumor specific antigens of methylcholanthrene induced sarcomas. Nature (Lond.) **204**, 846 (1964).

MOLOMUT, N.: Host induced alteration in strain specificity of Sarcoma I in mice. Reversibility of the change. Cancer Res. **18**, 906 (1958).

MOORE, T. L., KUPCHIK, H. Z., HANON, N., ZAMCHECK, N.: Carcinoembryonic antigen assay in cancer of the colon and pancreas and other digestive tract disorder. Amer. J. dig. Dis. **16**, 1 (1971).

MOORE, T., DHAR, P., ZAMCHECK, N., KUPCHICK, Z.: Canceroembryonic antigen (CEA) in diagnosis of digestive tract cancer. Ed. N. A. ANDERSON, J. COGGIN. In: Fetal and Embryonal Antigen in Cancer. **1**, 393 (1971).

MORKOV, J. K., SOKOLOV, J. N.: Successful surgical treatment of primary liver cancer. Chirurgia (USSR) **46**, 133 (1970) (in Russian).

MOULTON, M., STORER, J. B.: Maturation of the haemagglutination response in mice. Transplant. Bull. **30**, 150 (1962).

MUNA, N. M., MARCUS, S., SMART, C.: Detection of immunofluorescent of antibodies specific for human melanoma cells. Cancer (Philad.) **23**, 88 (1969).

MURPHY, J. B.: The lymphocyte in resistance to tissue grafting, malignant diseases and tuberculous infection. Monograph Rockefeller Institute **1**, (1926).

McBRIDE, C. M., BOWEN, J. M., DMOCHOWSKI, L.: Antinuclear antibodies in sera from patients with malignant melanoma. Surg. Forum **23**, 92 (1972).

McCALLION, D. J., TROTT, J. G.: Transient embryonic antigens in chick. J. Embryol. exp. Morph. **12**, 511 (1964).

McCALLION, D. J., LANGMAN, J.: An immunological study of the effect of brain extract on the developing neurons tissue in the chick embryo. J. Embryol. exp. Morph. **12**, 78 (1964).

McGREGOR, J.: Bone marrow origin of immunologically competent lymphocytes in the rat. J. exp. Med. **127**, 953 (1968).

McNEIL, C., LADLE, J. N., HELMICH, W. H., TRENTELMAN, E., WENTZ, M. W.: An antiserum to ovarian mucinous fluid with colon cancer specificity. Cancer Res. **29**, 1535 (1969).

NAIRN, R. C., RICHMOND, H. G., MacENTEGART, M. G., FOTHERGILL, J. E.: Immunological difference between normal and malignant cells. Brit. med. J. **2**, 1355 (1960).

NAIRN, R. C., FOTHERGILL, J. E., MACENTEGART, M. G., RICHMOND, H. G.: Loss of gastrointestinal specific antigen in neoplasia. Brit. med. J. **1**, 1191 (1962).

NAIRN, R. C., GHOSE, T., TANNENBERG, A. E.: Kidney specific antigen deletion in human renal carcinoma. Brit. J. Cancer **20**, 756 (1966).

NISHI, S.: Isolation and characterization of a human fetal alpha-globulin from the sera of fetuses and a hepatoma patient. Cancer Res. **30**, 2507 (1970).

NISHIOKA, M., IBATA, T., OHITA, K., HARADA, T., FUJITA, T.: Localization of alpha-fetoprotein in hepatoma tissue by immunofluorescence. Cancer Res. **32**, 162 (1972).

NORLAND, C. C., MAASS, E. G., KIRSUER, J. B.: Identification of colon carcinoma by immunofluorescent staining. Cancer (Philad.) **23**, 230 (1969).

OLDS, P.: An attempt to detect H-2 antigens on mouse eggs. Transplantation **6**, 478 (1968).

PALM, J., HEYNER, S., BRINSTER, R. L.: Differential immunofluorescence of fertilized mouse eggs with H-2 and non H-2 antibody. J. exp. Med. **133**, 1282 (1971).

PEARSON, G., FREEMAN, G.: Evidence suggesting a relationship between polyoma virus induced transplantation antigen and normal embryonic antigen. Cancer Res. **28**, 1665 (1968).

PEDERSON, K. O.: Fetuin, a new globulin isolated from serum. Nature (Lond.) **154**, 575 (1944).

PEREY, D. Y., COOPER, M. O., GOOD, R. A.: Lymphoepithelial tissue of the intesting and differentiation of antibody production. Science **161**, 265 (1968).

PLAYFAIR, J. H. L.: Strain differences in the immune response of mice. I. The neonatal response to sheep red blood cells. Immunology **15**, 35 (1968).

POKORNA, Z.: Induction of experimental autoimmune aspermatogenesis by immune serum fractions. Folia Biol. (Praha) **16**, 320 (1970).

POOL, E. H., DUNLAP, G. R.: Cancer cells in blood stream. Amer. J. Cancer **21**, 99 (1934).

PREHN, R. T.: Specific homograft tolerance induced by successive mating and implication concerning choriocarcinoma. J. nat. Cancer Inst. **25**, 883 (1960).

PREHN, R. T.: Tumor specific immunity to transplanted dibenzanthracene sarcomas. Cancer Res. **20**, 1614 (1960).

PREHN, R. T.: Specific isoantigenicity among chemically induced tumors. Ann. N.Y. Acad. Sci. **101**, 107 (1962).

PREHN, R. T.: The significance of tumor distinctive histocompatibility antigens. In: Crossreacting Antigen, p. 105. Ed.: J. J. TRENTIN. Baltimore: Williams and Wilkins 1967.

PURVES, L. R.: Serum alpha-fetoprotein. VIII. Serum levels during diethylnitroseamine poisoning of baboons. Int. J. Cancer **10**, 552 (1972).

PURVES, L. R., BERSOHN, I.: Radioimmunoassay of alpha fetoprotein. Proc. Sth. Afr. Ass. Path. p. 67. 1969.

PURVES, L. R., BERSOHN, I., GEDES, E. W.: Serum alpha-fetoprotein and primary cancer of the liver in man Cancer (Philad.) **25**, 1261 (1970).

PURVES, L. R., VAN DER MERVE, E., BERSOHN, I.: Variants of alpha-fetoprotein. Lancet **1970 II**, 464.

PURVES, L. R., MACNAB, M., GEDDES, E. *et al.*: Serum alpha fetoprotein and primary hepatic cancer. Lancet **1968 I**, 921.

PUTKONEN, T.: Über die gruppenspezifischen Eigenschaften verschiedener Körperflüssigkeiten. Acta Soc. Med. "Duodecim" A, 141 (1930).

PUZA, A., GOMBOS, A.: Acquired tolerance of skin homografts in dogs. Transplant. Bull. **5**, 30 (1958).

RAFF, M. C.: T and B lymphocytes in mice studied by using antisera against surface antigenic markers. Amer. J. Pathol. **65**, 467 (1971).

REYNOSO, G., CHU, T. M., HOLYOKE, D., *et al.*: Carcinoembryonic antigen in patients with different cancer. J. Amer. med. Ass. **220**, 361 (1972).

RHAMSDAHL, M. M., COX, I. S.: Immunofluorescent studies of antibodies against human malignant melanoma. Surg. Forum **201**, 126 (1969).

RIDLEY, A., CAVANAGH, J. B.: Lymphocytic infiltration in gliomas: evidence of possible host resistance. Brain **94**, 117 (1971).

ROANE, P. R., ROIZMAN, B.: Studies of the determinant antigens of viable cells II. Demonstration of altered antigenic reactivity of HEP-cells infected with herpes simplex virus. Virology **22**, 1 (1964).

ROMANOVSKY, A.: The effect of embryo specific and organ specific antisera on the developing frog embryos. Folia Biol. (Praha) **11**, 271 (1965).

RUOSLAHTI, E., SEPPÄLÄ, M., PIKKO, H., VUOPIO, P.: Studies of carcinofetal proteins. II. Biochemical comparison of alpha-fetoprotein from human fetuses and patients with hepatocellular cancer. Int. J. Cancer **8**, 283 (1971).

RUOSLAHTI, E., SEPPÄLÄ, M.: Normal and increased alphafetoprotein in neoplastic and non-neoplastic liver disease. Lancet **1972 II**, 278.

RUOSLAHTI, E., SEPPÄLÄ, M.: Studies of carcinofetal proteins: Physical and chemical properties of human alpha fetoprotein. Int. J. Cancer **7**, 218 (1971).

RUOSLAHTI, E., SEPPÄLÄ, M.: Studies of carcinofetal protein. III. Development of radioimmunoassay for a fetoprotein. Demonstration of a alpha-fetoprotein in serum of healthy human adults. Int. J. Cancer **8**, 374 (1971).

SAXEN, E., PENTTINEN, K.: Host factors in cell culture: Further studies on the growth controlling action of fresh human sera. J. nat. Cancer Inst. **26**, 1367 (1961).

SAXEN, E., PENTTINEN, I.: Host factors and cancer. Acta path. microbiol. Scand. **54**, 75 (1962).

SCHLESINGER, M.: Uterus of rodents as site for manifestation of transplantation immunity against transplantable tumors. J. nat. Cancer Inst. **28**, 927 (1962).

SCHLESINGER, M.: Serologic studies of embryonic and trophoblastic tissues of the mouse. J. Immunol. **93**, 255 (1964).

SCHINKEL, P. G., FERGUSON, K. A.: Skin transplantation in the fetal lamb. Aust. J. exp. Biol. med. Sci. **6**, 533 (1953).

SCHONE, E.: Über die Tumortransplantationen. Münch. med. Wschr. **51**, 1 (1906).

SEDALLIAN, J. P., JACOB, G.: Cytotoxic and cytolytic effect of mouse antiembryo sera on Ehrlich ascites cells. Nature (Lond.) **215**, 156 (1967).

SEHON, A. H.: The detection and nature of nonprecipitating antibodies in allergic sera. In: "Mechanism of hypersensitivity". Ed.: J. H. SHAFFE, G. A. LoGRIPPO, M. W. CHACE. Boston: Little, Brown and Co. 1959, p. 61.

SEPPÄLÄ, M., BAGSHAWE, K. D., RUOSLAHTI, E.: Radioimmunoassay of alphafetoprotein: A contribution to the diagnosis of choriocarcinoma and hydatiforme mole. Int. J. Cancer **10**, 478 (1972).

SEPPÄLÄ, M., TALBER, T., ENHOLM, C.: Studies on embryo specific proteins. Physiological characteristics of embryo specific alphaglobulin. Ann. Med. exp. Ferm. **45**, 16 (1967).

SEVER, J. L., HUEBNER, R. J., FABIYI, A.: Antibody responses in acute and chronic rubella. Proc. Soc. exp. Biol. N.Y. **122**, 513 (1966).

SEVER, J. L., BERENDES, H. W.: Abstr. Soc. Pediat. Res. april, 35 (1967).

SHEAHAN, D. G., HOROWITZ, S. A., ZAMCHECK, N.: Deletion of epithelial ABH isoantigens in primary gastric neoplasms and in metastatic cancer. Amer. J. dig. Dis. **16**, 961 (1971).

SILVERSTEIN, A. M.: Congenital syphilis and the timing of immunogenesis in the human fetus. Nature (Lond.) **194**, 196 (1962).

SILVERSTEIN, A. M., PRENDERGAST, R. A., KRANER, K. L.: Fetal response to antigenic stimulus. IV. Rejection of skin hemograft by the fetal lamb. J. exp. Med. **119**, 955 (1964).

SILVERSTEIN, A. M., PRENDERGAST, R. A., KRANER, K. Z.: Homograft rejection in the fetal lamb. The role of circulating antibody. Science **142**, 1172 (1964).

SILVERSTEIN, A. M., KRANER, K. L.: Studies on the ontogensis of immune response. In: Molecular and Cellular basis of Antibody Formation, p. 341. Ed.: J. STERZL. Praha: CSAV 1965.

SILVERSTEIN, A. M., PRENDERGAST, R. A., KRANER, K. L.: Fetal response to antigenic stimulus. IV. The rejection of skin homograft in the fetal lamb. J. exp. Med. **119**, 955 (1964).

SILVERSTEIN, A. M., UHR, J. W., KRANER, K. L., LUKES, R. J.: Fetal response to antigenic stimulus II. Antibody production by fetal lamb. J. exp. Med. **117**, 799 (1963).

SILVERSTEIN, A. M., LUKES, R. J.: Fetal response to antigenic stimulus. I. Plasmacellular and lymphoid reactions in the human fetus to intrauterine infection. Lab. Invest. **11**, 918 (1962).

SIMMONS, R. L., RUSSEL, P. S.: The histocompatibility antigens of fertilized mouse egg and trophoblast. Ann. N.Y. Acad. Sci. **129**, 35 (1967).

SIMMONS, R. L., RUSSEL, P. S.: Histocompatibility antigens in transplanted mouse eggs. Nature (Lond.) **208**, 698 (1965).

SIMMONS, R. L., RUSSEL, P. S.: The immunologic problem of pregnancy. Amer. J. Obstet. Gynec. **85**, 583 (1963).

SIMMONSEN, M.: Induced tolerance to heterologous cells and induced susceptibility to the virus. Nature (Lond.) **175**, 763 (1955).

SIMMONSEN, M.: Impact on developing embryo and newborn animal of adult homologous immunocompetent cells. Acta path. microbiol. scand. **40**, 480 (1957).

SINKOVICS, J. G., SHIRATO, E., CABINES, J. R., SHULTENBERGER, C. C.: Cytotoxic lymphocytes in Hodgkin disease. Brit. med. J. I, 172 **(1970)**.

SJOGREN, H. O.: Studies on the specific transplantation resistance against polyoma virus induced tumor. IV. Stability of the polyoma antigen. J. nat. Cancer Inst. **32**, 661 (1964).

SJOGREN, H. O.: Transplantation method as a tool for detection of tumor specific antigens. Prog. exp. Tumor Res. (Basel) **6**, 289 (1964).

SJOGREN, H. O., HELLSTROM, I., KLEIN, G.: Resistance of polyoma virus immunized mice against transplantation of established polyoma tumors. Exp. Cell Res. **23**, 204 (1961).

SJOGREN, H. O., JONSSON, N.: Resistance against transplantation of mouse tumors induced by Rous sarcoma virus. Exp. Cell Res. **32**, 618 (1964).

SJOGREN, H. O., HELLSTROM, I., BANSAL, S. C., HELLSTROM, K. E.: Suggestive evidence the "blocking" antibodies of tumors, bearing individuals are may be antigen antibody complexes. Proc. nat. Acad. Sci. (Wash.) **68**, 1372 (1971).

SMITH, J. B.: Alphafetoprotein in neoplastic and nonneoplastic conditions. In: Embryonal and Fetal Antigens in Cancer **1**, 305 (1971).

SMITH, J. B.: Occurrence of alpha fetoprotein in acute viral hepatitis. Int. J. Cancer **8**, 421 (1971).

SMITH, J. B., O'NEIL, R. T.: Alpha fetoprotein. Occurrence in geminal cell and liver malignancies. Amer. J. Med. **51**, 767 (1971).

SMITH, J. B., TODD, D.: Fetoglobulin and primary liver cancer. Lancet **1968 II**, 833.

SNELL, G. D.: Antigenic differences between the sperm of different inbred strains of mice. Science **100**, 272 (1944).

SNELL, G. D.: The genetic of transplantation. J. nat. Cancer Inst. **14**, 691 (1953).

SNELL, G. D.: The H-2 locus of the mouse: Observation and speculation concerning its comparative genetic and its polymorphism. Folia biol. (Praha) **14**, 335 (1968).

SOLOMON, J. B.: Fetal and neonatal immunology. p. 263. Amsterdam: North Holland Publishing Co. 1971.

SOUTHAM, C. M., BRUNSDHWIG, A., LEVIN, A. G., DIXON, Q. S.: Effect of leucocytes on transplantability of human cancer. Cancer (Philad.) **19**, 1743 (1966).

SPENCER, R. R.: Tumor immunity. J. nat. Cancer Inst. **2**, 317 (1942).

SPIRO, R. G.: Studies on fetuin, a glycoprotein of the fetal serum. J. biol. Chem. **235**, 2860 (1960).

SPIRO, M. J., SPIRO, R. G.: Composition of the peptide portion of fetuin. J. biol. Chem. **237**, 1507 (1962).

SPJUT, H. J.: Cancer cells in the pleural cavity. Cancer (Philad.) **11**, 1222 (1958).

STEINMULLER, D.: In: Transplantation of tissue and cells, p. 27. Ed.: BILLINGHAM, R. E., SILVERS, W. K. Philadelphia: Wistar Inst. Press 1961.

STEINMULLER, D.: Transplantation immunity in the newborn rat. I. The response at birth and maturation of response capacity. J. exp. Zool. **147**, 233 (1961).

STILLMAN, A., ZAMCHECK, N.: Recent advances in immunological diagnosis of digestive tract cancer. Amer. J. dig. Dis. **15**, 1003 (1970).

STONEHILL, E. H., BENDICH, A.: Retrogenic expression: The reappearance of embryonal antigens in cancer cells. Nature (Lond.) **228**, 370 (1970).

STEJRNSWARD, J., ALMGARD, L. E., FRANZEN, S., VON SCHREEB, T., WADSTROM, L. B.: Tumor distinctive cellular immunity in renal carcinoma. Clin. exp. Immunol. **6**, 963 (1970).

SVOBODA, J.: Analysis of acquired tolerance to the Rous sarcoma. Folia Biol. (Praha) **2**, 205 (1958).

TAL, C.: The nature of the cell membrane receptor for the agglutination factor present in the sera of tumor patients and pregnant women. Proc. nat. Acad. Sci. (Wash.) **54**, 1318 (1965).

TAL, C., DISHON, T., GROSS, J.: The agglutination of tumor cells in vitro by sera from tumor patients and pregnant women. Brit. J. Cancer **18**, 111 (1964).

TATARINOV, Y. S.: Presence of embryonal alpha globulin in the serum of patients with primary hepatocellular carcinoma. Vop. med. Klin. **1**, 90 (1964).

TATARINOV, Y. S.: Content of embryospecific alphaglobulin in blood serum of human fetus, newborn and adult man with primary cancer of the liver. Vop. med. Klin. **2**, 204 (1965).

TATARINOV, Y. S.: Variations in embryospecific alpha globulin in human blood sera in fetuses and the newborn. Nature (Lond.) **17**, 964 (1968).

TEVETHIA, S. S., RAPP, F.: Demonstration of new surface antigen in cells transformed by papova virus SV 40 in cytotoxic test. Proc. Soc. exp. Biol. (N.Y.) **12**, 455 (1965).

THOMPSON, D. M. P., KRUPEY, J., FREEDMAN, S. O.: The radioimmunoassay of circulating embryonic antigen of human digestive system. Proc. nat. Acad. Sci. (Wash.) **64**, 161 (1969).

TING, R. C.: Failure to induce transplantation resistance against polyoma tumor cells with syngeneic embryonic tissue. Nature (Lond.) **217**, 858 (1968).

TOOLAN, H. W.: Growth of humantumors in cortisone treated laboratory animals: The possibility of obtaining permanently transplantable human tumors. Cancer Res. **13**, 389 (1953).

TOOLAN, H. W.: Immunological responses elicited in the heterologous host by transplantable human tumors: Use of the conditioned rat as a test medium. Ann. N.Y. Acad. Sci. **69**, 830 (1957).

TOOLAN, H. W.: Permanently transplanted human tumors. Cancer Res. **17**, 418 (1957).

TOOLE, C. O., PERLMANN, P., UNSGARD, B., MOBERGER, G., EDSUNYR, F.: Cellular immunity to human urinary bladder carcinoma I. Correlation to clinical stage and radiotherapy. Int. J. Cancer **10**, 77 (1972).

TOOLE, O. C., PERLMANN, P., UNSGARD, B., ALMGARD, L. E., JOHANSSON, B., MOBERGER, G., EDSUNYR, F.: II. Effect of surgery and preoperative irradiation. Int. J. Cancer **10**, 92 (1972).

TROUILLAS, P.: Immunologie des tumeurs cèrèbrales: l'antigène carcinofétal glial. Ann. Inst. Pasteur **122**, 819 (1972).

TYAN, M. L.: Thymus. — Its role in maturation of fetal lymphoid precursors. Science **145**, 934 (1964).

TYAN, M. L.: Studies on the ontogeny of the mouse immune system. I. Cell bound immunity. J. Immunol. **100**, 535 (1968).

TYAN, M. L., CILE, L. J.: Development of transplantation antigens in the mouse embryo and trophoblasts. Transplant. Bull. **30**, 136 (1962).

TYAN, M. L., CILE, L. J.: Bone marrow as the major source of the potential immunological competent cells in the adult mouse. Nature (Lond.) **208**, 1223 (1965).

TYAN, M. L., CILE, L. J., HERZENBERG, L. A.: Fetal liver: A source of immunoglobulin-producing cells in the mouse. Proc. Soc. exp. Biol. (N.Y.) **124**, 1161 (1967).

TYZZER, E. E.: Tumor Immunity. J. Cancer Res. **1**, 125 (1916).

UEDA, Y., ITO, M., YAGAYU, I.: A specific surface antigen induced by Poxvirus. Virology **38**, 180 (1969).

UPHOFF, D. E.: Maternal modification of antigenicity: An immunological mechanism to ensure survival of mammalian fetuses. J. nat. Cancer Inst. **45**, 1189 (1970).

URIEL, J., NECHAUD, B., STANISLAWSKI-BIRENCWAJG, M.: Le diagnostic du cancer primaire du foie par méthode immunologique. Presse Méd. **76**, 1415 (1968).

URIEL, J., NECHAUD, B., STANISLAWSKI-BIRENCWAJG, M., MASSEYEFF, P., LEBLANC, L., QUEMMIN, C., LOISILIER, F., GRABAR, P.: Antigènes embryonaires et cancer du foie chez l'homme et association de l'alphafétoproteine sérique avec l'hépatoma primaire. C. R. Acad. Sci. (Paris) **265**, 75 (1967).

VANKY, F., STEJRNSWARD, J., NILSSON, V.: Cellular immunity to human sarcoma. J. nat. Cancer Inst. **46**, 1145 (1971).

VIERUCCI, A., GENAZZANI, A. R., MESSINA, A., FIORETTI, P.: Heterogeneity and distribution of human serum fetoproteins and character of the respective antibodies, p. 57. Milan: Excerpta Med. Int. Congress Series 183, 1968.

VIOSIN, P.: In: Mechanism of immunological tolerance. Ed.: M. HASEK. p. 67, Prague: Publ. House of Czechoslovack Acad. Sci. 1961.

VOJTISKOVA, M.: H-2d antigens on mouse spermatozoa. Nature (Lond.) **222**, 1293 (1969).

VOJTISKOVA, M., CHUTNA, J., RYCHLIKOVA, M., POKORNA, Z.: On the possible role of immunological tolerance in the prevention of autoimmune aspermatogenesis. Folia Biol. (Praha) **8**, 207 (1962).

VOJTISKOVA, M., POLASKOVA, M., POKORNA, Z.: Histocompatibility antigens on mouse spermatozoa. Folia Biol. (Praha) **15**, 322 (1969).

WATABE, E.: Early appearance of embryonic alpha globulin in rat serum during cancerogenesis with 4-dimethylazobenzene. Cancer Res. **31**, 1192 (1971).

WATME, A. L., MOORE, G. F., HATIBOGEN, I.: Cancer cell in thoracic lymph. Proc. Amer. Ass. Cancer Res. **3**, 72 (1959).

WEILER, E.: Die Änderung der serologischen Spezifizität von Leverzellen der Ratte während der Cancerogenese durch Dimethylazobenzol. Z. Naturforsch. **11** (b), 31 (1956).

Weiss, D. V., Fanklin, L. J., DeOme, K. B.: Acquisition of heightened resistance and susceptibility to spontaneous mouse mammary carcinoma of the original host. Cancer Res. **24**, 732 (1964).

Wiktor, T. J., Kuvert, E., Koprowski, H.: Immune lysis of rabies infected cells. J. Immunol. **101**, 1271 (1968).

Wissler, R. W., Barker, P. A., Flax, M. H., LaVia, M. F., Talmage, D. W.: A study of the preparation and effects of antitumor antibodies labelled with [131]I. Cancer Res. **16**, 76 (1956).

Willis, R. A.: The Borderland of Embryology and Pathology. London: Butterworths 1962.

Witebsky, E., Rose, N. R., Shulma, S.: Studies of normal and malignant tissue antigens. Cancer Res. **16**, 831 (1956).

Witebsky, E., Poplar, E.: Zur Methode des Nachweises carcinomaspezifischer Antigenfunktionen. Z. Immun-Forsch. **76**, 82 (1932).

Woglom, W. H.: Immunity of transplantable tumors. Cancer Rev. **4**, 129 (1929).

Wolffe, E., Wolff, E.: Culture organotypique de longe durée de deux tumeurs humaines du tube digestif. Europ. J. Cancer **2**, 93 (1966).

Wood, W. C., Morton, D. L.: Microcytotoxicity test: Detection in sarcoma patients of antibody cytotoxic to human sarcoma cells. Science **170**, 1318 (1970).

Woodruff, M. F.: Evidence of adaptation in homografts of normal tissue. Bull. Soc. int. Chir. **18**, 131 (1959).

Yachi, A., Matsura, Y., Carpenter, C. M., Hyde, L.: Immunochemical studies on human lung cancer antigens soluble in 50% saturated amonium sulphate. J. nat. Cancer Inst. **40**, 663 (1968).

Yaffe, O., Feldman, M.: Immunogenetic changes induced in tumors grown in radiation chimeras. J. nat. Cancer Inst. **23**, 133 (1959).

Yoon, I. L.: The eosinophil and gastrointestinal carcinomas. Amer. J. Surgery **97**, 195 (1959).

Zamcheck, N., Moore, T. L., Dhar, P., Kupchik, H. Z.: Summary of current status (March 1972) of clinical studies of carcinoembryonic antigens (CEA). Ed.: Anderson *et al.* In: Embryonic and Fetal Antigens in Cancer, Vol. **2**, 209 (1972).

Zamcheck, N., Moore, T. L., Dhar, P., Kupchik, H. Z.: Immunologic diagnosis and prognosis of human digestive tract cancer: Canceroembryoantigens. Med. Intell. **286**, 83 (1972).

Zeilmaker, G. H., Timmumans, A.: Development of mouse blastocytes under the kidney capsule of irradiated rats. Transplant. Bull. **7**, 437 (1969).

Zilber, L. A., Abelev, G. I.: The virology and immunology of cancer, p. 383: Pergamon Press 1968.

Zilber, L. A., Krjukova, I. N., Narcissov, N. V., Biriulina, T. I.: The serological differentiation of extracts of Rous sarcoma and normal tissue. Probl. Oncol. (N.Y.) **4**, 285 (1958).

Zilber, L. A.: Specific tumor antigens. Advanc. Cancer Res. **6**, 291 (1958).

Zilber, L. A., Abelev, G. I., Avenirova, Z. A., Engelgardt, N. V., Bajdakova, Z. L.: Dokl. Akad. Nauk SSSR, Otd. Biol. **124**, 927 (1959).

Subject Index

Allogeneic graft 1
Alphafetoprotein, diagnostic value 41, 46, 47
— in nontumor diseases 30
—, properties 36
—, species specificity 29
Antigens, organ specific 4
—, transplantation 1
—, tumor specific 5, 7, 19
—, — — T(CF) 22
—, Y-linked 4
Autoimmune disease 8
Autotransplantation 1

Canceroembryoantigen, alphafetoprotein 29
—, cell surface related 24
—, — —, human 25, 27
—, digestive tract, antibodies against 46
—, — —, aminoacid composition 36
—, — —, chemical composition 39
—, — —, cell localisation 32, 38
—, — —, diagnostic value 42
—, — —, gastric cancer 33
—, — —, localisation 35
—, — —, in nondigestive tract tumors 43
—, — —, non tumor diseases 44, 45
—, — —, prognostic value 45
—, — —, properties 38
—, — —, *in vitro* production 38
—, immunodiffusion 51
—, immunofluorescence 52
—, immunotherapy 49

Canceroembryoantigen, methods of detection 51
—, properties 35, 29
—, purification 53
—, radioimmunoassay 52
—, viral tumors 26, 28

Egg, antigenicity 11
Ehrlich ascites tumor 24
Embryo, antigenicity 13
—, immune reactivity 14
—, mother fetus relation 13
Enhancement 6, 8

Heterograft(xeno-) 1
Histocompatibility locus 3

Immunological reaction 6
Inbred strains 1

Microorganisms, cell membrane related 4

Parabiosis, embryonic 9
Paralysis, immunologic 9

Secondary response 6, 8
Sperm, antigenicity 12
Syngeneic graft 1

Tolerance 6, 14
Transplantation antigens, modification 6
— —, mutation 6

Recent Results in Cancer Research

Sponsored by the Swiss League against Cancer. Editor in chief: P. Rentchnick, Genève

1 SCHINDLER, R.: Die tierische Zelle in Zellkultur. Geb. DM 18,—; US $ 7.00

2 Neuroblastomas — Biochemical Studies. Edited by C. BOHUON, (Symposium). Cloth DM 18,—; US $ 7.00

3 HUEPER, W. C.: Occupational and Environmental Cancers of the Respiratory System. Cloth DM 37,—; US $ 14.30

4 GOLDMAN, L.: Laser Cancer Research. Cloth DM 18,—; US $ 7.00

5 METCALF, D.: The Thymus. Its Role in Immune Responses, Leukaemia Development and Carcinogenesis. Cloth DM 26,—; US $ 10.10

6 Malignant Transformation by Viruses. Edited by W. H. KIRSTEN, (Symposium). Cloth DM 35,—; US $ 13.50

7 MOERTEL, CH. G.: Multiple Primary Malignant Neoplasms. Their Incidence and Significance. Cloth DM 20,—; US $ 7.70

8 New Trends in the Treatment of Cancer. Edited by L. MANUILA, S. MOLES, and P. RENTCHNICK. Cloth DM 35,—; US $ 13.50

9 LINDENMANN, J., and P. A. KLEIN: Immunological Aspects of Viral Oncolysis. Cloth DM 20,—; US $ 7.70

10 NELSON, R. S.: Radioactive Phosphorus in the Diagnosis of Gastrointestinal Cancer. Cloth DM 17,—; US $ 6.60

11 FREEMAN, R. G., and J. M. KNOX: Treatment of Skin Cancer. Cloth DM 17,—; US $ 6.60

12 LYNCH, H. T.: Hereditary Factors in Carcinoma. Cloth DM 26,—; US $ 10.10

13 Tumours in Children. Edited by H. B. MARSDEN and J. K. STEWARD. Cloth DM 79,—; US $ 30.50

14 ODARTCHENKO, N.: Production Cellulaire Erythropoiétique. Relié DM 31,—; US $ 12.00

15 SOKOLOFF, B.: Carcinoid and Serotonin. Cloth DM 26,—; US $ 10.10

16 JACOBS, M. L.: Malignant Lymphomas and Their Management. Cloth DM 20,—; US $ 7.70

17 Normal and Malignant Cell Growth. Edited by R. J. M. FRY, M. L. GRIEM, and W. H. KIRSTEN (Symposium). Cloth DM 56,80; US $ 21.90

18 ANGLESIO, E.: The Treatment of Hodgkin's Disease. Cloth DM 24,—; US $ 9.30

19 BANNASCH, P.: The Cytoplasm of Hepatocytes during Carcinogenesis. Electron- and Lightmicroscopical Investigations of the Nitrosomorpholine-intoxicated Rat Liver. Cloth DM 32,—; US $ 12.40

20 Rubidomycin. A new Agent against Cancer. Edited by J. BERNARD, R. PAUL, M. BOIRON, C. JACQUILLAT, and R. MARAL. Cloth DM 48,—; US $ 18.50

21 Scientific Basis of Cancer Chemotherapy. Edited by G. MATHÉ (Symposium). Cloth DM 28,—; US $ 10.80

22 KOLDOVSKÝ, P.: Tumor Specific Transplantation Antigen. Cloth DM 24,—; US $ 9.30

23 FUCHS, W. A., J. W. DAVIDSON, and H. W. FISCHER: Lymphography in Cancer. With contributions by G. JANTET and H. RÖSLER. Cloth DM 76,—; US $ 29.30

24 HAYWARD, J. L.: Hormones and Human Breast Cancer. An Account of 15 Years Study. Cloth DM 34,—; US $ 13.10

25 ROY-BURMAN, P.: Analogues of Nucleic Acid Components. Mechanisms of Action. Cloth DM 28,—; US $ 10.80

26 Tumors of the Liver. Edited by G. T. PACK and A. H. ISLAMI. Cloth DM 56,—; US $ 21.60

27 SZYMENDERA, J.: Bone Mineral Metabolism in Cancer. Cloth DM 32,—; US $ 12.40

28 MEEK, E. S.: Antitumour and Antiviral Substances of Natural Origin. Cloth DM 16,—; US $ 6.20

29 Aseptic Environments and Cancer Treatment. Edited by G. MATHÉ (Symposium). Cloth DM 22,—; US $ 8.50

30 Advances in the Treatment of Acute (Blastic) Leukemias. Edited by G. MATHÉ (Symposium). Cloth DM 38,—; US $ 14.70

31 DENOIX, P.: Treatment of Malignant Breast Tumors. Indications and Results. Cloth DM 48,—; US $ 18.50

32 NELSON, R. S: Endoscopy in Gastric Cancer. Cloth DM 48,—; US $ 18.50

33 Experimental and Clinical Effects of L-Asparaginase. Edited by E. GRUNDMANN and H. F. OETTGEN (Symposium). Cloth DM 58,—; US $ 22.40

34 Chemistry and Biological Actions of 4-Nitroquinoline 1-Oxide. Edited by H. ENDO, T. ONO, and T. SUGIMURA. Cloth DM 36,—; US $ 13.90

35 PENN, I.: Malignant Tumors in Organ Transplant Recipients. Cloth DM 24,—; US $ 9.30

36 Current Concepts in the Management of Lymphoma and Leukemia. Edited by J. E. ULTMANN, M. L. GRIEM, W. H. KIRSTEN, and R. W. WISSLER (Symposium). Cloth DM 48,—; US $ 18.50

37 CHIAPPA, S., R. MUSUMECI, and C. USLENGHI: Endolymphatic Radiotherapy in Malignant Lymphomas. With contributions by G. BONADONNA, B. DAMASCELLI, G. FAVA, F. PIZZETTI, U. VERONESI. Cloth DM 48,—; US $ 18.50

38 KOLLER, P. C.: The Role of Chromosomes in Cancer Biology. Cloth DM 48,—; US $ 18.50

39 Current Problems in the Epidemiology of Cancer and Lymphomas. Edited by E. GRUNDMANN and H. TULINIUS (Symposium). Cloth DM 58,—; US $ 22.40

40 LANGLEY, F. A., A. C. CROMPTON: Epithelial Abnormalities of the Cervix Uteri. Cloth DM 58,—; US $ 22.40

41 Tumours in a Tropical Country. A Survey of Uganda (1964—1968). Edited by A. C. TEMPLETON. Cloth DM 72,—; US $ 27.80

42 Breast Cancer: A Challenging Problem. Edited by M. L. GRIEM, E. V. JENSEN, J. E. ULTMANN, and R. W. WISSLER (Symposium). Cloth DM 48,—; US $ 18.50

43 Nomenclature, Methodology and Results of Clinical Trials in Acute Leukemias. Edited by G. MATHÉ, P. POUILLART, and L. SCHWARZENBERG (Symposium). Cloth DM 58,—; US $ 22.40

44 Special Topics in Carcinogenesis. Edited by E. GRUNDMANN (Symposium). Cloth DM 58,—; US $ 22.40

45 KOLDOVSKÝ, P.: Carcinoembryonic Antigens. Cloth DM 38,—; US $ 14.70

Special Supplement: Biology of Amphibian Tumors. Edited by M. MIZELL. Cloth DM 86,—; US $ 33.20

In Production

46 Diagnosis and Therapy of Malignant Lymphoma. Edited by K. MUSSHOFF (Symposium). Cloth DM 62,—; US $ 23.90

Prices are Subject to change without notice

47 Investigation and Stimulation of Immunity in Cancer Patients. Edited by G. MATHÉ and R. WEINER (Symposium)

48 Platinum Compounds in Cancer Chemotherapy. Edited by T. A. CONNORS and J. J. ROBERTS (Symposium)

49 Complications of Cancer Chemotherapy. Edited by G. MATHÉ and R. K. OLDHAM (Symposium)

MIX
Papier aus verantwortungsvollen Quellen
Paper from responsible sources
FSC® C105338

If you have any concerns about our products,
you can contact us on
ProductSafety@springernature.com

In case Publisher is established outside the EU,
the EU authorized representative is:
Springer Nature Customer Service Center GmbH
Europaplatz 3, 69115 Heidelberg, Germany

Printed by Libri Plureos GmbH
in Hamburg, Germany